SpringerBriefs in Psychology

SpringerBriefs in Child Development

Beth Troutman

Integrating Behaviorism and Attachment Theory in Parent Coaching

Springer

Beth Troutman
Department of Psychiatry
University of Iowa Carver College
of Medicine
Iowa City
Iowa
USA

ISSN 2192-8363 ISSN 2192-8371 (electronic)
Sub ISSN 2192-838X Sub ISSN 2192-8398 (electronic)
SpringerBriefs in Psychology
ISBN 978-3-319-15238-7 ISBN 978-3-319-15239-4 (eBook)
DOI 10.1007/978-3-319-15239-4

Library of Congress Control Number: 2015933015

Springer Cham Heidelberg New York Dordrecht London

Springer is a brand of Springer International Publishing
Springer International Publishing is part of Springer Science+Business Media (www.springer.com)

In memory of my parents,
Betty McClure Troutman and Gary Troutman

Preface

"There is nothing more practical than a good theory." (Lewin 1952)
"Each investigator begins with the paradigm of choice and discovers its inadequacies." (Patterson 1982)

This book is for providers and trainees (infant and early childhood mental health therapists, home visitors, pediatricians, nurses, and other early interventionists) who advise and guide parents of infants, toddlers, and young children (0–8). The goal is to help providers address concerns about the parent-child relationship, the child's emotional development, and the child's behavior problems. This book provides a framework for early interventionists to incorporate the most recent research on behavioral and attachment approaches to parenting into their practice. There is a particular emphasis on addressing the types of concerns most likely to bring families to the attention of providers—conflictual parent-child relationships, harsh parenting or maltreatment, and child conduct problems.

Over the past 50 years, two different theoretical models have guided parenting advice and intervention—behaviorism and attachment theory. Each of these models has spawned rich programs of research and staunch supporters. These two traditions have also led to sometimes conflicting recommendations regarding how to best respond to infants/young children and sometimes conflicting views of "positive parenting". With an increasing focus on research-informed interventions in work with families, these traditions have also led to competing claims regarding research support for various positive parenting approaches.

I speak both behaviorism and attachment theory. Although this sounds silly, there is some truth to it. Behaviorism and attachment theory have their own terminology which complicates communication between researchers and therapists in these two traditions and makes it difficult for providers to evaluate competing viewpoints.

As a clinical child psychologist whose interest in the field of infant and early childhood mental health began in the 1970s, I came of age as a parent-child therapist/researcher during the growth of interventions based on behaviorism and attachment theory. I find value in both theoretical orientations. My clinical training includes training in behavioral interventions for disruptive behavior, behavioral interventions for anxiety disorders, parent coaching interventions, and interventions based on attachment theory. My research incorporates concepts from social learning theory, attachment theory, and temperament theory.

The goal of Part I is making research about behaviorism and attachment theory more accessible to providers. Chapter 1 provides an overview of how behaviorists view parent-child interactions and outcomes research on evidence-based behavioral parenting interventions for young children with disruptive behavior and families at risk for maltreatment. There is a particular emphasis on outcomes research for the behavioral parenting approach I have been disseminating for the past decade, Parent-Child Interaction Therapy (PCIT). Chapter 2 provides an overview of attachment theory and outcomes research on interventions based on attachment theory. There is a particular emphasis on attachment theory-based approaches that influence my framework for working with families of young children. Chapter 3 summarizes some of the areas of disagreement between these two traditions and begins to explore how the two theories may complement each other.

Part II is the "to do" part of the book. The goal of Part II is providing therapists with a framework for integrating behaviorism and attachment theory when coaching parents of young children. If you're more of a doer, you may want to dive into Part II of the book first and read the earlier chapters only as questions arise about theory, assessments, or methodology. (Of course, if you're a doer, you're probably one of those readers who skips the preface.) Chapter 4 lays out the rationale for using parent coaching to address problematic parent-child interactions and a framework for incorporating attachment theory and research into parent coaching. Chapters 5, 6, 7, and 8 discuss tailoring parent coaching to different patterns of attachment.

Acknowledgements

This book owes its birth to the students and community providers I have trained. Your questions about research and your commitment to providing high quality parenting interventions spurred me to write a book describing my approach to parent coaching and the research that informs my approach. This book also belongs to the PCIT therapists who attended my presentation on *Using Observations of Attachment to Inform Parent-Child Interaction Therapy Coaching* at the 13th annual Parent-Child Interaction Therapy Conference in Los Angeles in 2013 and to Anthony Urquiza, Susan Timmer, and Emma Girard who facilitated the presentation. Your interest in knowing more about an attachment-informed approach to PCIT coaching made me realize there was more interest in this topic than I'd thought and, since few of you were likely to travel to Iowa for workshops, I was going to have to write a book in order to communicate my ideas. (Thanks to Marta Shinn for being one of the few Californians willing to brave Iowa weather and become an adopted Iowan. Go Hawks!).

I am indebted to Brenda Hollingsworth and Mary Mohrhauser for seeing my emerging capacities to train community providers before I truly saw them myself. Your faith in my abilities to train Iowa providers got this started and your enthusiasm and faith that I will figure out the next step keeps it going.

I owe a special thanks to participants in the attachment for PCIT therapists workshops and conference calls, especially those of you who attended the first attachment workshop for PCIT therapists and continue to promote it (Dawn Combites, Desiree Cunningham-Loggins, Leesa Dzuris, Kami Guzman, Mary Haskins, Jess O'Bleness, Sandy Pelzer, Kelli Slagle Radermacher, Nancy Wallace, and Claire Wofford). Your excitement and ability to see the potential of combining attachment and behavioral parent coaching approaches contributed to me continuing down this path. The kind words of first readers of early versions of this manuscript (Kelly Pelzel, Tania Cargo, Sue Morgan, and LeAnn Lape-Brinkman) provided me the encouragement I needed to try and get my ideas down on paper. Thanks to my editor Garth Haller for shepherding me through the process of actually getting my ideas in print and coming up with a title without a colon.

For me, John Knutson, Alan Sroufe, Betty Carlson, Dymphna van den Boom, June Sroufe, Cheryl McNeil, Kent Hoffman, and Ellen Moss embody the best of the behavioral and attachment theory traditions. I feel fortunate to have learned behavioral parenting interventions and attachment theory from such excellent teachers. I am grateful to have learned behavioral parent coaching from John Knutson. Without this parent coaching experience, I doubt I would have come to appreciate behavioral parenting interventions. I am grateful to Alan Sroufe and Betty Carlson for teaching me to code attachment classifications from the Strange Situation Procedure. Your quiet patience as the first teachers to help me view interactions through an attachment lens is a model for how teachers can serve as a secure base. Once I learned to view parent-infant relationships through this lens, there was no going back. I am grateful to Dymphna van den Boom for sharing my passion for irritable babies, teaching me to code maternal sensitive responsiveness to the attachment signals of irritable babies, and teaching me her attachment theory-based intervention for irritable infants. Our discussions about coding, attachment theory, temperament, and academic camps are among my best training experiences and speak volumes about your brilliant mind. Your willingness to take the time for these discussions as a busy young faculty member speaks to your generous heart. I am grateful to June Sroufe for teaching me to code the Adult Attachment Interview (AAI). You turned what I thought might be a tedious coding enterprise into one of the most enlightening trainings I have ever experienced and provided a model for creating a safe space for discussion and reflection. I am grateful to Cheryl McNeil for mentoring me in training community therapists in PCIT and for making several trips to Iowa and Nebraska to co-train with me. Our discussions about attachment theory and behaviorism during dinners and long drives across Iowa helped me think about how to explain attachment theory and research to behaviorists. I am grateful to Kent Hoffman for training in Circle of Security (COS), expanding my thinking about states of mind, and providing a holding environment to reflect on my own shark music. Our discussions about attachment theory and behaviorism helped me articulate the differences between these two approaches. I am grateful to Ellen Moss for teaching me to code attachment classifications in the modified Strange Situation Procedure for pre-schoolers. The opportunity to view attachment in goal-directed partnerships and learn about your efforts to train community providers in attachment and Relationship Intervention for Parents provided the missing ingredients for my training program. It was such a joy to meet someone else who spoke both attachment and behaviorism and to discuss how PCIT and attachment coaching approaches might complement each other.

It "takes a village" to do research on attachment theory. I have been fortunate to be a part of two such villages. My own village of research assistants, students, and colleagues who assisted with the infant emotional development study (Christian Aliaga, Steve Arndt, Callie Berry, Linsey Blair, Jamie Bulleri, Michelle Cardi, Christina Durham Weeks, Leanne Florke, Christina Franklin, Jennifer Gianone, Kate Hancock, Altier Juarez, Sarah Lowery, Erika Luttennegger, E. Imani Mitchell-Burrell, Allison Momany, Tracy Moran Vozar, Susan Ryan, Donna Stewart, Lisa Tibey, and Brooke van Horne) and Kristen Casper's and Remi Cadoret's village of researchers interested in adult attachment and adoption (Steve Arndt, Bruce Pfohl, Rob Philibert, and Becca Yucuis). I also benefited from being a member of Betsy Momany's village of researchers interested in the needs of children in foster care – especially her willingness to prioritize making a difference over getting reports written.

I learned much from the infants, children, and parents who have participated in my research, training, and clinical services. As a grandmother at an in-home visit once told me "each baby is as unique as each snowflake". The opportunity to learn from each family's unique strengths and struggles makes my work continually interesting and challenging. Your willingness to share your parenting experiences and let me hang out with your babies and young children makes my work continually enjoyable.

This book would not have been possible without the love and support of my husband, Ralph Johnson. Thank you for making me laugh, making me question, and teaching me about ethology, the music of Leonard Cohen, and how to write an NIH grant. You are the kite, the string, and the spool.

Contents

About the Author

Beth Troutman, Ph.D., is a Clinical Professor in Psychiatry at the University of Iowa Carver College of Medicine. Her teaching, research, and clinical work has focused on improving parent-child interactions for more than 30 years. She has had a foot in more than one theoretical camp since graduate school, conducting research on parenting self-efficacy, temperament, and attachment theory and disseminating Parent-Child Interaction Therapy (PCIT), a behavioral model for improving parenting.

Part I
Two Models for Viewing Parent-Child Interactions: Behaviorism and Attachment Theory

Chapter 1
Viewing Parent-Child Interactions Through the Lens of Behaviorism

"Coercive behaviors are maintained by both positive and negative reinforcement." (Patterson 1982)

Standing in line at the grocery store behind a harried looking mother pushing a shopping cart with a 2-year-old boy and a cart full of groceries, you watch the 2-year-old reach out and grab a pack of cookies from the shelf[1]. *His mother says "No. Cookies will just make you more hyper. Put the cookies back on the shelf." He shakes his head no and clutches the cookies to his chest. She pries the cookies from his chubby little hands and returns them to the shelf. He emits a full-pitched scream, slaps at her, and yells "Bad Mommy". His mother moves out of his reach while he continues to scream and yell at her. The shopper in line ahead of the mother turns around and says to the boy "It sounds like someone is having a bad day. Maybe you're hungry." Neither the mother nor child respond to the shopper but the mother takes a fruit snack out of her purse and offers it to her son. He knocks the fruit snack out of her hand and uses this brief diversion to grab the pack of cookies off the shelf again. As the shopper in line ahead finishes her purchase, the mother pushes her cart forward and begins putting items on the conveyer belt. She snatches the much coveted cookies out of her son's hands and adds them to the pile of items on the conveyer belt. Her son begins wailing again. She turns to him and says "Stop it. You can have the cookies. I have to pay for them first." The clerk hurriedly scans the cookies and hands them to the mother. The mother says "Thank you" to the clerk and quickly returns the cookies to her son. The 2-year-old quiets immediately while you, the clerk, and the other shoppers breathe a sigh of relief. The toddler gives you a beatific smile as he proudly holds up his pack and says "Cookies!".*

[1] This is a fictional account written to illustrate application of behavioral principles to parent-child interactions.

B. Troutman, *Integrating Behaviorism and Attachment Theory in Parent Coaching*, SpringerBriefs in Psychology, DOI 10.1007/978-3-319-15239-4_1

Positive and Negative Reinforcement of Behaviors

From the perspective of behaviorism, the parent-child interaction described in the above vignette reflects the parent and child's reinforcement history—i.e. certain behaviors have been strengthened and weakened through reinforcement and punishment. Of particular interest to early interventionists is how the parent and child reinforce and punish each other's behavior. Positive reinforcement refers to a stimulus that increases the probability a behavior will occur again (i.e. strengthen the behavior) when it occurs following the behavior. The other type of reinforcement in operant conditioning is negative reinforcement. Negative reinforcement is often confused with punishment. Although both negative reinforcement and punishment involve aversive stimuli, they have the opposite effect on behavior. Negative reinforcement involves strengthening a behavior by *removing* an aversive stimulus contingent upon the behavior.

To the casual observer, the most obvious aspect of the shopping vignette at the beginning of this chapter is the mother positively reinforcing the child's misbehavior by giving him the cookies, increasing the likelihood he will engage in the same misbehavior the next time they go to the store. (We might also predict the store manager will continue to put small packs of cookies on the aisle before the checkout since he is positively reinforced for placing them there by an increase in cookie sales.) Negative reinforcement is less obvious but may be operating in the above example as well. The mother is negatively reinforced for giving her son the cookies by the termination of his aversive behavior. Since "giving in" to his demands when his misbehavior escalates has been reinforced, the mother is more likely to give in to his demands the next time his misbehavior escalates.

*On the other hand, the shopping experience has been so aversive the mother has been punished for taking her son shopping, increasing the likelihood she will leave him with his father the next time she goes to the store. In the above exchange, the mother and child use both verbal and nonverbal behavior in their attempts to influence each other's behavior. We are struck by the number of aversive behaviors they exhibit towards each other, an interactional sequence described by Patterson (*1982*) as a "coercive exchange". Conflicts escalate as the members of the dyad use increasingly coercive methods in an attempt to control the other person's behavior.*

It is easy for parents to fall into a "reinforcement trap" (Patterson 1982) when disciplining young children. Observational research of parents' interactions with their young children indicates parents' aversive responses (i.e. reprimands and negative nonverbal responses) to a young child's noncompliance increase compliance in the short-run (Owen et al. 2012). This means parents receive immediate reinforcement for responding to noncompliance with reprimands and negative nonverbal responses. The problem is, over time, parent-child interactions may become increasingly aversive for both parent and child as each member of the dyad is positively and negatively reinforced for the use of aversive behaviors. In some dyads, this may escalate to the point where the parent becomes physically abusive, leading providers to look to behavioral interventions to intervene in this coercive cycle.

Behavioral Assessment of Parent-Child Interactions

Much of the behavioral research on parent-child interactions is based on standardized situations where a parent and child are observed interacting in a clinic or laboratory setting. Typically, the setting looks like a play room and the parent and child are observed using a one-way mirror or surveillance camera. Examples of standardized situations where parent-child interactions are observed include: "unstructured play" (parent is told to play with their child as they would at home), "child-led play" (parent is told to follow the child's lead in play), "structured play" (parent is given specific tasks for child to complete using play materials) "parent-led play" (parent is told to have the child follow their lead in the play), and "clean-up" (parent is told to have the child clean up the toys) (Eyberg et al. 2013; Mash and Johnston 1983; Robinson and Eyberg 1981).

During unstructured or child-led play, children referred for disruptive behavior exhibit higher frequencies of touching their parent, whining, yelling, and pretend play verbalizations and lower frequencies of praising their parent and exhibiting a positive response to their parent's praise compared to community samples (Forster et al. 1990; Mash and Johnston 1983; Robinson and Eyberg 1981; Speltz et al. 1995). Parents of children referred for disruptive behavior criticize their child more, give their child more direct commands, and praise their child less during child-led play (Aragona and Eyberg 1981; Robinson and Eyberg 1981; Speltz et al. 1995). Contrary to a common perception that parents of children with disruptive behavior fail to address the child's misbehavior, parents of children referred for behavior problems are *more* likely to respond to their child's deviant behavior (rather than ignoring it) than parents of nonreferred children (Speltz et al. 1995). During a clean-up situation, children referred for disruptive behavior engage in more deviant behavior and obey a smaller percentage of parent commands than nonreferred children (Speltz et al. 1995).

Overall, research on the frequencies of parent and child behaviors in dyads referred for clinical services paint a picture of interactions that are often unrewarding and unpleasant for both members of the dyad. When viewing conflictual parent-child interactions, there is a strong pull to "side" with either the parent or child. Both "sides" have compelling arguments. When viewed from the parent's perspective, it would be much easier to praise and refrain from criticizing a child who was praising you, complying with your commands, and not engaging in disruptive behavior. When viewed from the child's perspective, it would be easier to comply with commands if your parent was less demanding, less critical, and paid more attention to your positive behavior.

Positive Parenting Skills—Behavioral Perspective

Parenting interventions based on behaviorism dominate the research literature on psychosocial interventions for disruptive behavior problems in young children. The majority of these interventions are based on interventions developed by Patterson or Hanf in the 1960s (Hanf 1969; Hanf and Kling 1973) resulting in a number of similarities between the various behavioral parent training interventions.

From a behavioral perspective, parental attention is a powerful reinforcer that can be used to shape the child's behavior. Positive parenting skills include attending to the child's appropriate behavior and ignoring inappropriate behavior. Most misbehavior is addressed using differential reinforcement of other behavior. That is, parents are taught to attend to behaviors that are the "positive opposite" of or incompatible with misbehavior.

Behavioral interventions use shaping or positive reinforcement for successive approximations. That is, when a child is learning a new skill, he is positively reinforced for behaviors that are "baby steps" towards the target behavior.

In the hypothetical shopping vignette, the mother would be encouraged to take her child on a brief shopping trip where she focused on praising his positive behavior and only purchased a couple of items in order to shape more appropriate behavior during shopping trips. She would be encouraged to praise the child for sitting quietly in the shopping cart, being a good helper, and "looking with their eyes" (rather than their hands).

In evidence-based behavioral interventions, aversive consequences such as reprimands and time-out from positive reinforcement are viewed as necessary to reduce disruptive behavior but are used much less frequently than positive reinforcement (Owen et al. 2012).

Several behavioral parenting interventions for young children evolved from a two stage in vivo parent coaching model originally developed by Connie Hanf (Hanf 1969; Hanf and Kling 1973). In this model, parents are coached through a bug-in-the-ear to use differential social attention to modify their child's behavior during the first stage of treatment. The differential social attention skills are taught in the context of child-led play. Since most children are fairly well-behaved in a situation where they have their parent's undivided attention while playing, parents have the opportunity to learn to attend to their child's positive, appropriate behavior. In the second stage of treatment, parents are taught to teach their child to follow directions (compliance training) by rewarding the child for compliance and using aversive consequences (warning and time-out from positive reinforcement) for noncompliance. This stage of treatment is also introduced in the context of a play session (parent-led play) so the parent has an opportunity to practice the behavioral parenting skills being introduced and the child has an opportunity to learn to comply in a low stress situation. One of the relatively unique aspects of Hanf's approach is the use of behavioral coding to determine whether parents meet behavioral criteria indicating acquisition of specific behavioral skills.

Widely-used behavioral parenting interventions that have evolved from Hanf's approach include Incredible Years (Webster-Stratton 1982), Helping the Noncompliant Child (Forehand and McMahon 1981; McMahon and Forehand 2003), and Parent-Child Interaction Therapy (PCIT) (Eyberg and Funderburk 2011; Hembree-Kigin and McNeil 1995; McNeil and Hembree-Kigin 2010; Urquiza et al. 2011). The Incredible Years parent training approach is a group intervention where standard videotapes of parent-child interactions are used to teach parents behavioral parenting skills. Studies demonstrating the efficacy of the Incredible Years approach to behavioral parent training were first published in the 1980s and evidence built rapidly (Webster-Stratton 1982). A meta-analysis of 50 studies of Incredible Years parent training indicates this approach is effective in improving prosocial behavior and decreasing disruptive behavior for children with clinically significant levels of disruptive behavior or at risk of developing disruptive behavior (Menting et al. 2013).

The two approaches that have maintained Hanf's emphasis on in vivo parent coaching, coding parent-child interactions each session, and having parents meet specific behavioral performance criteria are Helping the Noncompliant Child (Forehand and McMahon 1981; McMahon and Forehand 2003) and PCIT (Eyberg and Funderburk 2011). During in vivo parent coaching sessions, parents wear a bug-in-the-ear and are observed and coached through a one-way mirror while interacting with their child.

In-Session Coding of Behavioral Parenting Skills/ Behavioral Performance Criteria

In Helping the Noncompliant Child, parents must acquire and demonstrate several different behavioral parenting skills during child-led play (McMahon and Forehand 2003). Parents are required to meet behavioral performance criteria for each skill before learning the next skill. In the first phase, parents are taught to attend (i.e. describe the child's behavior). The parent must demonstrate 20 attends and two or fewer commands and questions during 5 min of child-led play before learning the next skill. The next skill parents are taught is rewarding their child's behavior (i.e. praising the child's behavior and giving nonverbal positive touches such as hugs and pats on the back). Behavioral performance criteria for this phase is giving at least 10 rewards, at least 20 attends plus rewards, and two or fewer commands and questions during 5 min of child-led play. After the parent demonstrates a high rate of positive attention by meeting these behavioral performance criteria, the parent is taught to ignore inappropriate child behavior. Behavioral performance criteria for this phase is ignoring 70 % of the child's inappropriate behavior (inappropriate behavior is predefined by the therapist and parent).

The first phase of compliance training in Helping the Noncompliant Child involves teaching parents to give clear, direct commands (alpha commands). To meet the behavioral performance criteria for this phase of treatment, the parent must give an average of 10 alpha commands in 5 min of parent-led play and 75 % or more of commands given must be alpha commands. Behavioral performance criteria for the next phase of treatment, giving consequences for compliance and noncompliance, is giving the child a reward (praise or nonverbal positive touch) after at least 60 % of the child's compliance with commands during 5 min of parent-led play. The child must also meet behavioral performance criteria during this phase of treatment, compliance with 75 % of parent commands.

In PCIT, specific behavioral performance critieria that must be met by parents are referred to as "mastery criteria" (Eyberg and Funderburk 2011; McNeil and Hembree-Kigin 2010; Urquiza et al. 2011). Although several studies of PCIT demonstrate significant reductions in disruptive behavior even when parents are not required to meet mastery criteria (Eisenstadt et al. 1993; Nieter et al. 2013; Nixon et al. 2003), most recent studies of PCIT to address disruptive behavior require parents meet mastery criteria for positive parenting skills during child-led play before moving to the compliance training phase.

Early versions of PCIT required parents demonstrate 20–25 positive verbal parenting responses following the child's appropriate behavior (i.e. behavioral descriptions, reflections, and/or labeled praises) during 5 min of child-led play prior to moving to the compliance training phase of treatment (Hembree-Kigin and McNeil 1995; Schuhmann et al. 1998). Current versions of PCIT require parents demonstrate 30 positive verbal parenting responses to the child's appropriate behavior (i.e. 10 behavioral descriptions, 10 reflections, and 10 labeled praises) and no more than three questions, commands, or criticisms during 5 min of child-led play prior to moving to the next phase of treatment (Eyberg and Funderburk 2011; McNeil and Hembree-Kigin 2010; Urquiza et al. 2011). Parent's behavioral performance criteria for the compliance training phase of PCIT are giving effective commands 75 % of the time (i.e. alpha commands) and following through with appropriate consequences after 75 % of alpha commands (i.e. labeled praise for compliance, warning for noncompliance, time-out for positive reinforcement for noncompliance following warning) (Eyberg and Funderburk 2011).

There are no head-to-head studies comparing different behavioral parent training protocols. Thus, interventionists often use factors other than research outcomes in choosing a specific behavioral parenting intervention to implement. I have implemented several different behavioral parenting protocols and prefer approaches that utilize in vivo parent coaching through a bug-in-the-ear such as Helping the Noncompliant Child (McMahon and Forehand 2003) and PCIT (Eyberg and Funderburk 2011; McNeil and Hembree-Kigin 2010; Urquiza et al. 2011). These approaches give me the opportunity to observe the parent and child interactions in the moment and tailor my coaching.

The specific behavioral parenting intervention I have focused on implementing, disseminating, and training community providers in for the past decade is PCIT. Information about PCIT has become more accessible during the past decade as it has moved out of Universities and into communities. Additional information on PCIT training at the University of Iowa is available at this web site: http://www.medicine.uiowa.edu/psychiatry/parentchildinteractiontherapy/.

The University of California at Davis has an excellent web site about their PCIT training program where you can complete a free webinar on PCIT for Traumatized Children (PCIT-TC), download PCIT-TC forms in English and Spanish, and download behavioral coding (Dyadic Parent-Child Interaction Coding System (DPICS)) manuals in English and Spanish: http://pcit.ucdavis.edu/. Information about PCIT training and dissemination is also available at the PCIT International web site where you can purchase a PCIT protocol and DPICS manual: http://www.pcit.org/. For therapists interested in learning more about PCIT, I also highly recommend Parent-Child Interaction Therapy, Second Edition (McNeil and Hembree-Kigin 2010).

As shown in Table 1.1, PCIT is clearly effective at reducing disruptive behavior. Parent's ratings of disruptive behavior tend to show greater improvement than behavioral assessments of disruptive behavior. Parent ratings may be more sensitive to change due to differences between the types of assessments (e.g. behavioral assessments may be too brief to show significant changes). The significant changes in parent ratings of disruptive behavior indicate PCIT leads to changes in the parent's perceptions of the child as well as changes in the child's behavior.

As shown in Table 1.2, parents participating in PCIT exhibit significant increases in their use of positive behavioral parenting skills such as praising and describing their child's behavior and significant decreases in their use of criticism, commands, and questions. Table 1.2 also displays the relatively high percentage of families who drop out of PCIT prior to completing treatment. Although the significant drop-out rate in PCIT is a concern, this rate fails to capture my experience providing PCIT to families and consulting on PCIT with community providers. I find many of the families who drop out prior to completing treatment display improved parent-child interactions and significant reductions in disruptive behavior, often to the nonclinical range. Thus, although the parents are not willing to continue treatment in order to meet the predetermined behavioral performance criteria, I do not consider these families to be treatment failures.

Child outcomes associated with PCIT in child welfare/child maltreatment populations are shown in Table 1.3. Parent outcomes and drop-out rates are shown in Table 1.4. As shown in Table 1.3, children with a history of maltreatment or at risk for maltreatment who participate in PCIT with either their foster parent (McNeil et al. 2005; Timmer et al. 2006) or primary caregiver (Chaffin et al. 2011; Chaffin et al. 2004; Galanter et al. 2012; Nieter et al. 2013; Thomas and Zimmer-Gembeck 2011, 2012) demonstrate significant improvement in disruptive behavior, anxiety, and depression. Somewhat surprisingly, given the primary focus on changing the *parent's* behavior in studies where the parent had maltreated the child or was at risk of maltreating the child, only two of these six studies required the parent meet mastery criteria (Galanter et al. 2012). In the Chaffin et al. (2004) study, only 30% of physically abusive parents participating in PCIT met mastery criteria.

As shown in Table 1.4, PCIT reduces re-reports for abuse although rates remain high (17–47%). Research indicates children and parents referred from the child welfare system show improvement without parents meeting the PCIT mastery criteria established for parents of children with disruptive disorders (Chaffin et al. 2004, 2011; McNeil et al. 2005; Nieter et al. 2013; Thomas and Zimmer-Gembeck 2011,

Table 1.1 Child outcomes in studies of parent-child interaction therapy (PCIT) in children with disruptive behavior

Population	Model	Behavioral assessment of child behavior	Parent report of child behavior	Reference
Preschool-aged children referred for conduct problems (United States) $N=10$	PCIT	*Compliance (CLP, PLP, & CU)* PCIT $d=1.8$	*Disruptive behavior (ECBI)* PCIT $d=-2.6$	McNeil et al. 1991
Preschool-aged children referred for behavior problems (United States) $N=31$	PCIT[a]	*Compliance/deviant behaviors (CLP, PLP, & CU)* PCIT $d=1.8/-0.64$	*Disruptive behavior (ECBI)* PCIT $d=-2.7$	Eisenstadt et al. 1993
Preschool-aged children referred for disruptive behavior (United States) $N=64$	PCIT WL	*Compliance with mother*[b] Pre PCIT: 23 % Post PCIT: 47 % Compliance with father[b] Pre PCIT: 27 % Post PCIT: 45 %	*Mother rating of disruptive behavior (ECBI)* PCIT $d=-1.5$ WL $d=-0.1$ *Father rating of disruptive behavior (ECBI)* PCIT $d=-1.2$ WL $d=-0.2$	Schuhmann et al. 1998
Preschool-aged children referred for behavior problems (Australia) $N=92$	PCIT[c] ABB PCIT[d]	*Compliance/deviant behaviors with mother* (CLP, PLP, & CU) PCIT $d=0.74/-0.49$ ABB PCIT $d=0.53/-0.26$ WL $d=0.55/-0.74$	*Mother rating of disruptive behavior (ECBI)* PCIT $d=-2.03$ ABB PCIT $d=-1.68$ WL $d=-1.21$ *Father rating of disruptive behavior (ECBI)* PCIT $d=-1.0$ ABB PCIT $d=-1.1$ WL $d=-0.5$	Nixon et al. 2003
Young children referred for behavior problems (United States) $N=70$; 72	PCIT	Not reported	*Disruptive behavior (ECBI)* PCIT $d=-1.0$ *Exernalizing (CBCL)* PCIT $d=-1.0$ *Internalizing (CBCL)* PCIT $d=-1.0$	Timmer et al. 2006

Table 1.1 (continued)

Population	Model	Behavioral assessment of child behavior	Parent report of child behavior	Reference
Preschool-aged children with diagnoses of both oppositional defiant disorder and mental retardation (United States) $N=30$	PCIT	*Compliance (PLP & CU)* PCIT $d=1.41$ WL $d=-.43$	*ECBI* PCIT $d=-2.0$ WL $d=-0.9$	Bagner and Eyberg 2007
Children referred to community providers for behavior problems. (United States) $N=154$	PCIT	Not reported	*ECBI* $d=-1.2$ *TSCYC post-traumatic stress total* $d=-0.7$ *TSCYC dissociation* $d=-0.7$ *TSCYC anger* $d=-1.1$	Pearl et al. 2012
Children referred for behavior problems (United States) $N=120$	clinic and in-home PCIT	Not reported	*ECBI* PCIT completers (clinic and in-home) $d=-0.9$	Lanier et al. 2011

PCIT parent-child interaction therapy, *CLP* child-led play, *PLP* parent-led play, *CU* clean up, *d* Cohen's *d*, *ECBI* Eyberg Child Behavior Inventory, *ABB PCIT* abbreviated PCIT, *WL* wait list, *TSCYC* trauma symptom checklist for young children

[a]half of sample received parent-directed interaction prior to child-directed interaction

[b]*d* could not be calculated as SD was not reported

[c]In the version of PCIT used in this study parents were coached during five sessions of child-led play and seven sessions of parent-led play

[d]In the abbreviated version of PCIT used in this study five coaching sessions were alternated with 5 30 min telephone consultations

Table 1.2 Drop-out rates and parent outcomes in studies of parent-child interaction therapy (PCIT) with children with disruptive behavior

Population	Model	Drop-out rate	Behavioral assessment of parent behavior	Reference
Preschool-aged children referred for conduct problems (United States) $N=10$	PCIT	0%	Not reported	McNeil et al. 1991
Preschool-aged children referred for behavior problems (United States) $N=31$	PCIT[a]	35%	Not reported	Eisenstadt et al. 1993
Preschool-aged children referred for disruptive behavior (United States) $N=64$	PCIT WL	PCIT: 41% WL: 26%	*Mother % praise (CLP, PLP, & CU)* PCIT $d=2.1$ WL $d=0.4$ *Mother % criticism (CLP, PLP, & CU)* PCIT $d=-1.1$ WL $d=-0.5$ *Mother % behavioral description (CLP, PLP, & CU)* PCIT $d=7.0$ WL $d=0.9$ *Father % praise (CLP, PLP, & CU)* *PCIT $d=2.2$* *WL $d=0$* *Father % criticism (CLP, PLP, & CU)* PCIT $d=-1.3$ WL $d=-0.4$ *Father % behavioral description (CLP, PLP, & CU)* PCIT $d=1.7$ WL $d=0$	Schuhmann et al. 1998
Preschool-aged children referred for behavior problems (Australia) $N=92$	Strd PCIT Ab PCIT WL	Strd PCIT: 23% Ab PCIT: 13% WL: 6%	*Mother praise (CLP, PLP, & CU)* Strd PCIT $d=2.0$ Ab PCIT $d=1.2$ WL $d=0.5$ *Mother criticism (CLP, PLP, & CU)* Strd PCIT $d=1.1$ Ab PCIT $d=0.6$ WL $d=0.2$	Nixon et al. 2003

Table 1.2 (continued)

Population	Model	Drop-out rate	Behavioral assessment of parent behavior	Reference
Young children referred for behavior problems (United States) $N=70$	PCIT	53 %	Not reported	Timmer et al. 2006
Preschool-aged children with diagnoses of both Oppositional Defiant Disorder and Mental Retardation (United States) $N=30$	PCIT	PCIT: 33 % WL: 20 %	*Praise + Reflection + Behavior Description (CLP)* PCIT $d=1.9$ WL $d=0.4$ *Question + Command + Criticism (CLP)* PCIT $d=-2.7$ WL $d=-0.8$	Bagner and Eyberg 2007
Children referred to community providers for behavior problems. (United States) $N=154$	PCIT	67 %	*Praise + Reflection + Behavior Description (CLP)* $d=2.9^{b}$	Pearl et al. 2012
Children referred for behavior problems (United States) $N=120$	PCIT In-Home PCIT	PCIT: 72 % In-Home PCIT: 66 %	Not reported	Lanier et al. 2011

PCIT parent-child interaction therapy, *CLP* child-led play, *PLP* parent-led play, *CU* clean up, *d* Cohen's *d*, *Strd PCIT* standard PCIT, *Ab PCIT* abbreviated PCIT, *WL* wait list

[a]half of sample received parent-directed interaction prior to child-directed interaction

[b]data on subsample of 21 parents

Table 1.3 Child outcomes in studies of parent-child interaction therapy (PCIT) in child welfare/maltreatment populations

Population	Model	Behavioral assessment of child behavior	Parent report of child behavior	Reference
Physically abusive parent and physically abused child	ME+PCIT[a] ME+EPCIT[a] CS	Not reported	*Externalizing (CBCL)* ME+PCIT d=−1.9 ME+EPCIT d=−3.6 CS d=−0.9 *Internalizing (CBCL)* ME+PCIT d=−3.1 ME+EPCIT d=−1.8 CS d=−1.2	Chaffin et al. 2004
Foster parents of a young foster child with disruptive behavior (United States) N=30	Group PCIT[b] (2 day workshop)	Not reported	*ECBI* Group PCIT d=−0.8	McNeil et al. 2005
Foster parents of a foster child with disruptive behavior (United States) N=54; 65	PCIT	Not reported	*ECBI* PCIT d=−1.2 *Externalizing (CBCL)* PCIT d=−0.5 *Internalizing (CBCL)* PCIT d=−0.6	Timmer et al. 2006
Maltreating parent (physically abusive and/or neglectful) and maltreated child (United States) N=192	ME+PCIT[a] CSOR+PCIT[a] CSOR+CS ME+CS	Not reported	Not reported	Chaffin et al. 2011
Mothers identified as having a history of maltreating their child or at high risk of maltreating their child (Australia) N=150	PCIT		*ECBI* PCIT d=−1.3 *Externalizing (CBCL)* PCIT d=−0.8 *Internalizing (CBCL)* PCIT d=−0.6	Thomas and Zimmer-Gembeck 2011

Table 1.3 (continued)

Population	Model	Behavioral assessment of child behavior	Parent report of child behavior	Reference
Families identified as high-risk of or engaged in child maltreatment (Australia) $N=151$	Short PCIT [c] WL	Not reported	*ECBI* Ab PCIT $d=-0.4$ WL $d=-0.2$	Thomas and Zimmer-Gembeck 2012
Families identified as being at-risk for child maltreatment (United States) $N=83$	In-home PCIT	*Compliance (PLP)* In-home PCIT $d=1.5$	*ECBI* In-home PCIT $d=-1.2$	Galanter et al. 2012
Parents referred for child maltreatment (54 %) and/or assistance managing child behavior problems (children aged 2–8) (United States) $N=27$	Group PCIT [d]	Not reported	*ECBI* Group PCIT $d=-0.9$	Nieter et al. 2013

ME+PCIT motivational enhancement orientation and PCIT, *ME+EPCIT* motivational enhancement orientation and enhanced PCIT (individualized enhanced services target parental depression or substance abuse, family problems, marital problems, or domestic violence), *CS* community services, *d* Cohen's *d* (calculated on pre to post changes), *CBCL* child behavior checklist (Achenbach 2000), *CSOR+PCIT* community services orientation and PCIT; *CSOR+CS* community services orientation and community services, ME+CS motivational enhancement orientation and community services, ECBI eyberg child behavior inventory, *Ab PCIT* abbreviated PCIT (progression from Child-Directed Interaction (CDI) phase to Parent-Directed Interaction (PDI) phase occurs after 6 to 8 sessions regardless of assessment of parent's behavioral parenting skills, *WL* wait list, *CLP* child-led play, *PLP* parent-led play

[a]In the version of PCIT used in this study, parents were not required to meet specified mastery criteria for behavioral parenting skills

[b]In the version of PCIT used in this study, coding of parents' behavioral parenting skills was not conducted and parents were not required to meet specified mastery criteria in Child-Directed Interaction (CDI) prior to learning Parent-Directed Interaction (PDI)

[c]Short PCIT. (Parent is not required to meet mastery criteria and treatment concludes after a maximum of 12 coaching sessions have been conducted.)

[d]In the group version of PCIT used in this study parents received three CDI coaching sessions and five PDI coaching sessions. Families did not have to meet mastery criteria for CDI in order to progress to PDI

Table 1.4 Drop-out rate and parent outcomes in studies of parent-child interaction therapy (PCIT) in child welfare/maltreatment populations

Population	Model	Drop-out rate	Parent behavior	Reference
Physically abusive parent and physically abused child	ME+PCIT[a] ME+EPCIT[a] CS	Not reported	*Re-report for physical abuse*[b] ME+PCIT: 19% ME+EPCIT: 36% CS: 49% *Negative parent behaviors* ME+PCIT $d=-3.7$ ME+EPCIT $d=-2.8$ CS $d=1.7$ *Positive parent behaviors* ME+PCIT $d=1.0$ ME+EPCIT $d=1.3$ CS $d=-0.4$	Chaffin et al. 2004
Foster parents of a young foster child with disruptive behavior. (United States) $N=30$	Group PCIT[b] (2 day workshop)	10%	Not reported	McNeil et al. 2005
Foster parents of a foster child with disruptive behavior (United States) $N=75$	PCIT	52%	Not reported	Timmer et al. 2006
Maltreating parents and maltreated child (United States) $N=192$	ME+PCIT CSOR+PCIT CSOR+CS ME+CS	20%	*Re-report for maltreatment*[c] ME+PCIT: 29% CSOR+PCIT: 47% CSOR+CS: 41% ME+CS: 34%	Chaffin et al. 2011
Mothers identified as high risk of maltreating their child or engaged in child maltreatment (Australia) $N=150$	PCIT	PCIT: 58%	*Notification to child protection* PCIT completers: 17% PCIT drop-outs: 43% Praise: $d=1.9$ Desc. & Ref.: $d=1.2$ Questions $d=-1.7$ Commands $d=-0.6$	Thomas and Zimmer-Gembeck 2011
Families identified as high risk of maltreating their child or engaged in child maltreatment (Australia) $N=151$	Short PCIT[d] WL	Short PCIT[d]: 32%	*% praise (CLP)* Short PCIT[d] $d=1.3$ WL $d=0.1$ *% criticism (CLP)* Short PCIT $d=-0.3$ WL $d=-0.2$	Thomas and Zimmer-Gembeck 2012

Table 1.4 (continued)

Population	Model	Drop-out rate	Parent behavior	Reference
Families identified as being at risk for child maltreatment (United States) $N=83$	In-home PCIT	35 %	*Positives (CLP)* In-home PCIT $d=1.9$	Galanter et al. 2012
Parents referred for child maltreatment (54 %) and/or assistance managing child behavior problems (United States) $N=27$	Group PCIT[e]	37 %	*Prosocial (CLP)* $d=1.2$	Nieter et al. 2013

PCIT parent-child interaction therapy, d=Cohen's d (calculated on pre to post changes), *ME+PCIT* motivational enhancement orientation and PCIT, *ME+EPCIT* motivational enhancement orientation and enhanced PCIT (individualized enhanced services target parental depression or substance abuse, family problems, marital problems, or domestic violence), *CS* community services, *CSOR+PCIT* community services orientation and PCIT, *CSOR+CS* community services orientation and community services, *ME+CS* motivational enhancement orientation and community services, *Desc* descriptions, *Ref* reflections, *WL* wait list, *CLP* child-led play, *PLP* parent-led play

[a]In the version of PCIT used in this study, parents were not required to meet specified mastery criteria,

[b]median follow-up is 850 days

[c]median follow-up is 904 days

[d]Short PCIT. (Parent is not required to meet mastery criteria and treatment concludes after a maximum of 12 coaching sessions have been conducted.)

[e]In the group version of PCIT used in this study parents received three CDI coaching sessions and five PDI coaching sessions. Families did not have to meet mastery criteria for CDI in order to progress to PDI

2012). Based on these results and the high rate of attrition in PCIT, a recent article argues for using a short version of PCIT without mastery criteria requirements with parents referred from the child welfare system (Thomas and Herschell 2013). Despite these findings and recommendations, I require foster parents and parents referred for abusing or neglecting their child meet mastery criteria for Child-Directed Interaction (CDI) prior to teaching them Parent-Directed Interaction (PDI) skills. My rationale is: (1) It is important for children who have been maltreated to experience highly positive child-led play with primary caregivers. (2) It is important for primary caregivers of children who have been maltreated to overlearn attending to the child's appropriate, prosocial behavior since children who have been maltreated are more likely to become engaged in coercive exchanges with their caregivers. (3) It is important for caregivers who parent children who have been maltreated to experience the increase in self-efficacy that results from achieving a difficult goal (Troutman et al. 2012). (4) It is important for caregivers who have a history of becoming physically abusive or withdrawing from interactions in response to the child's misbehavior to overlearn attending to the child's positive, prosocial behavior since they are likely to resort to old patterns of behavior with their child when under stress.

Conclusions

Research on interventions based on a behavioral view of parent-child interactions indicates teaching parents to attend to their child's positive behavior, ignore minor misbehavior, give clear, direct commands, and use time-out from positive reinforcement for noncompliance and aggression, is associated with reductions in children's disruptive behavior, anxiety, and trauma symptoms in families with a child referred for disruptive behavior or at risk for disruptive behavior. Among parents with a history of maltreating their child or at risk of maltreating their child, behavioral parenting interventions are associated with a reduction in reports for maltreatment, although rates remain high. The shortcoming of behavioral parenting interventions is the large number of families who drop out prior to completing treatment.

References

Achenbach, T. R. L. (2000). *Manual for the ASEBA preschool forms & profiles*. Burlington: ASEBA.

Aragona, J., & Eyberg, S. (1981). Neglected children: Mothers' report of child behavior problems and observed verbal behavior. *Child Development, 52*(2), 596–602.

Bagner, D., & Eyberg, S. (2007). Parent-child interaction therapy for disruptive behavior in children with mental retardation: A randomized controlled trial. *Journal of Clinical Child and Adolescent Psychology, 36*(3), 418–429.

Chaffin, M., Silovsky, J., Funderburk, B., Valle, L., Brestan, E., Balachova, T., Jackson S., Lensgraf J., & Bonner, B. (2004). Parent-child interaction therapy with physically abusive parents:

Efficacy for reducing future abuse reports. *Journal of Consulting and Clinical Psychology, 72*(3), 500–510.

Chaffin, M., Funderburk, B., Bard, D., Valle, L., & Gurwitch, R. (2011). A combined motivation and parent-child interaction therapy package reduces child welfare recidivism in a randomized dismantling field trial. *Journal of Consulting and Clinical Psychology*. doi:10.1037/a0021227.

Eisenstadt, T. H., Eyberg, S. M., McNeil, C. B., Newcomb, K., & Funderburk, B. (1993). Parent-child interaction therapy with behavior problem children: Relative effectiveness of two stages and overall treatment outcomes. *Journal of Clinical Child Psychology, 22,* 42–51.

Eyberg, S., & Funderburk, B. (2011). *Parent-child interaction therapy protocol*. Gainesville: PCIT International, Inc.

Eyberg, S., Nelson, M., Ginn, N., Bhuiyan, N., & Boggs, S. (2013). *Dyadic parent-child interaction coding system (DPICS)* (4th ed.). Gainesville: PCIT International, Inc.

Forehand, R., & McMahon, R. (1981). *Helping the noncompliant child: A clinician's guide to parent training*. New York: The Guilford.

Forster, A., Eyberg, S., & Burns, L. (1990). Assessing the verbal behavior of conduct problem children during mother-child interactions: A preliminary investigation. *Child & Family Behavior Therapy, 12*(1), 13–22.

Galanter, R., Self-Brown, S., Valente, J., Dorsey, S., Whitaker, D., Bertuglia-Haley, M., & Prieto, M. (2012). Effectiveness of parent-child interaction therapy delivered to at-risk families in the home setting. *Child & Family Behavior Therapy, 34,* 177–196.

Hanf, C. (1969). *A two-stage program for modifying maternal controlling during mother-child (M-C) interaction*. Paper presented at the Western Psychological Association, Vancouver, BC.

Hanf, C., & Kling, J. (1973). *Facilitating parent-child interaction: A two-stage training model*. Oregon: University of Oregon Medical School.

Hembree-Kigin, T., & McNeil, C. (1995). *Parent-child interaction therapy*. New York: Plenum Press.

Lanier, P., Kohl, P., Benz, J., Swinger, D., Mousette, P., & Drake, B. (2011). Parent-child interaction therapy in a community setting: Examining outcomes, attrition, and treatment setting. *Research on Social Work Practice, 21*(6), 689–698.

Mash, E., & Johnston, C. (1983). The prediction of mothers' behavior with their hyperactive children during play and task situations. *Child & Family Behavior Therapy, 5,* 1–14.

McMahon, R., & Forehand, R. (2003). *Helping the noncompliant child: Family-based treatment for oppositional behavior* (2nd ed.). New York: Guilford.

McNeil, C., & Hembree-Kigin, T. (2010). *Parent-child interaction therapy* (2nd ed.). New York: Springer.

McNeil, C., Eyberg, S., Eisenstadt, T. H., Newcomb, K., & Funderburk, B. (1991). Parent-child interaction therapy with behavior problem children: Generalization of treatment effects to the school setting. *Journal of Clinical Child and Adolescent Psychology, 20*(2), 140–151.

McNeil, C., Herschell, A., Gurwitch, R., & Clemens-Mowrer, L. (2005). Training foster parents in parent-child interaction therapy. *Education & Treatment of Children, 28*(2), 182–196.

Menting, A., de Castro, B., & Matthys, W. (2013). Effectiveness of the incredible years parent training to modify disruptive and prosocial child behavior: A meta-analytic review. *Clinical Psychology Review, 33,* 901–913.

Nieter, L., Thornberry, T., & Brestan-Knight, E. (2013). The effectiveness of group parent-child interaction therapy with community families. *Journal of Child and Family Studies, 22,* 490–501.

Nixon, R., Sweeney, L., Erickson, D., & Touyz, S. (2003). Parent-child interaction therapy: A comparison of standard and abbreviated treatments for oppositional defiant preschoolers. *Journal of Consulting and Clinical Psychology, 71*(2), 251–260.

Owen, D., Slep, A., & Heyman, R. (2012). The effect of praise, positive nonverbal response, reprimand, and negative nonverbal response on child compliance: A systematic review. *Clinical Child and Family Psychology Review, 15,* 364–385.

Patterson, G. (1982). *Coercive family process*. Eugene: Castalia Publishing Company.

Pearl, E., Thieken, L., Olafson, E., Boat, B., Connelly, L., Barnes, J., & Putnam, F. (2012). Effectiveness of community dissemination of parent-child interaction therapy. *Psychological Trauma: Theory, Research, Practice, and Policy, 4*(2), 204–213.

Robinson, E., & Eyberg, S. (1981). The dyadic parent-child interaction coding system: standardization and validation. *Journal of Consulting and Clinical Psychology, 49*(2), 245–250.

Schuhmann, E., Foote, R., Eyberg, S., Boggs, S., & Algina, J. (1998). Efficacy of parent-child interaction therapy: Interim report of a randomized trial with short-term maintenance. *Journal of Clinical Child Psychology, 27*(1), 34–45.

Speltz, M., DeKlyen, M., Greenberg, M., & Dryden, M. (1995). Clinic referral for oppositional defiant disorder: Relative significance of attachment and behavioral variables. *Journal of Abnormal Child Psychology, 23*(4), 487–507.

Thomas, R., & Herschell, A. (2013). Parent-child interaction therapy: A manualized intervention for the therapeutic child welfare sector. *Child Abuse & Neglect, 37,* 578–584.

Thomas, R., & Zimmer-Gembeck, M. (2011). Accumulating evidence of parent-child interaction therapy in the prevention of child maltreatment. *Child Development, 82*(1), 177–192.

Thomas, R., & Zimmer-Gembeck, M. (2012). *Parent-child interaction therapy: An evidence-based treatment for child maltreatment.* Child Maltreatment, *17*(3), 253–266.

Timmer, S., Urquiza, A., & Zebell, N. (2006). Challenging foster caregiver-maltreated child relationships: The effectiveness of parent-child interaction therapy. *Children and Youth Services Review, 28,* 1–19.

Troutman, B., Moran, T., Arndt, S., Johnson, R., & Chmielewski, M. (2012). Development of parenting self-efficacy in mothers of infants with high negative emotionality. *Infant Mental Health Journal, 33*(1), 45–54.

Urquiza, A., Zebell, N., McGrath, J., & Whitten, L. (2011). *Course of treatment manual for PCIT-TC*. Davis: University of California at Davis. http://pcit.ucdavis.edu.

Webster-Stratton, C. (1982). Teaching mothers through videotape modeling to change their children's behavior. *Journal of Pediatric Psychology, 7*(3), 279–294.

Beth Troutman is a Clinical Professor in Psychiatry at the University of Iowa Carver College of Medicine. Her teaching, research, and clinical work has focused on improving parent-child interactions for more than 30 years. She has had a foot in more than one theoretical camp since graduate school, conducting research on parenting self-efficacy, temperament, and attachment theory and disseminating Parent-Child Interaction Therapy (PCIT), a behavioral model for improving parenting.

Chapter 2
Viewing Parent-Child Interactions Through the Lens of Attachment Theory

> *"The child who is attached to his mother, if he is secure in this attachment, does not need to maintain constant proximity or contact with her. He is content to move away, as long as he knows that she is there. He can even leave the room on his own initiative, and his aplomb in so doing is sometimes in sharp contrast to his consternation when his secure base gets up and moves off." (Ainsworth 1967)*

Three-year-olds Amy, Betty, and Cathy[1] *arrive at the park with their mothers. Amy and Betty run to the swings while their mothers settle onto nearby park benches. Cathy tugs at her mother's sleeve and whines to go to the slide. Her mother sits down on a bench, pulls out her cell phone, and says "You go play." Cathy continues to tug and whine saying "Come with me." Her mother sighs, puts her cell phone in her purse, and follows Cathy to the slide. Once at the slide, Cathy says "It's too high. I'm scared. I want to swing." Amy and Betty jump out of the swings simultaneously, landing hard, falling forward, and bumping heads. Amy gets up, brushes herself off, and walks to the slide. Betty starts to cry and walks towards her mother. Her mother opens her arms with a sympathetic expression asking "Did you get the wind knocked out of you?". Betty nods her head mutely and leans in to give her mother a hug. After they hug, Betty says "I want to go on the slide." Betty's mother says "okay" and Betty runs to the slide.*

Attachment Theory

In their quest to develop a science of relationships, John Bowlby and Mary Ainsworth developed ways of talking about attachment that differ from the informal use of these terms (Ainsworth 1967; Ainsworth et al. 1978; Bowlby 1969).

[1] This is a fictional account written to illustrate an attachment view of parent-child interactions.

B. Troutman, *Integrating Behaviorism and Attachment Theory in Parent Coaching*, SpringerBriefs in Psychology, DOI 10.1007/978-3-319-15239-4_2

For example, while a casual observer of the hypothetical playground scene might describe Cathy as "too attached" or Amy as "not attached", attachment theorists would focus on their ***patterns*** *of attachment. When viewed through the lens of attachment theory, Betty exhibits a balance between exploration and attachment described as consistent with secure attachment. Although Cathy exhibits more proximity-seeking and contact-maintaining behaviors than Betty and Amy, she would not be described as "more attached". Similarly, Amy would not be described as "unattached" because she fails to seek comfort when hurt. Instead, their patterns of interacting with their mothers would be viewed as patterns of attachment that maximize their chances of maintaining proximity to their mothers.*

Development of Attachment Theory

In order to view child-parent relationships through the lens of attachment theory, it helps to understand how attachment theory developed and how concepts central to attachment theory and research are operationalized. Attachment theory began as the study of the impact of separation and loss. John Bowlby, a child psychiatrist who studied with child psychoanalyst Melanie Klein, began developing his ideas about attachment theory and documenting the impact of separation from caregivers on children in England during the 1940s—a time of significant loss and disruption in attachment relationships due to World War II.

Bowlby's colleague, James Robertson, who was trained as a social worker and psychoanalyst, described three phases young children went through when separated from their caregivers—protest, despair, and detachment (Robertson 1953b). Robertson's films of young children's responses to separation from their primary caregiver are compelling and undeniable (e.g. (Robertson 1953a, 1971)). James Robertson and his wife, Joyce Robertson, who was also trained as a social worker and psychoanalyst, had the important insight that the reactions of children following separation from caregivers was impacted by the quality of the attachment relationship prior to the separation as well as the quality of substitute caregiving (Robertson and Robertson 1989). Consistent with their training as social workers, the Robertsons campaigned tirelessly to ameliorate the impact of separation from primary caregivers. For example, they provided foster care for children in their home and vividly describe the children's reaction to separation as well as how they supported them during the separation. James Robertson also worked with hospitals to raise awareness about the impact of separating young children from their caregivers and change policies that limited parents' visits when their children were hospitalized.

Mary Ainsworth, a colleague of Bowlby and Robertson who was trained as a psychologist, was also interested in documenting how the quality of the attachment relationship prior to separation impacted the reaction to separation. She also recognized the need to determine whether a child was attached to a caregiver in order to evaluate the impact of separation. With this goal in mind, she began a naturalistic, observational study of 26 mothers and infants in Uganda where, she had been told, infants were briefly separated from their mothers at the time of weaning (Ainsworth 1967). Although the majority of infants were not separated for weaning, Ainsworth's observations and extensive field notes provided important insights about the development of attachment. She identified several different infant behaviors (listed in Table 2.1) indicating an infant had become attached to a specific caregiver. Ainsworth noted that in addition to being indicators of attachment, these behaviors also facilitated the further development of the attachment relationship. For example, expressing delight and greeting her mother when she walks in the room is an indication an infant is attached to her mother but it also contributes to a positive attachment relationship by increasing the mother's positive feelings towards the

Table 2.1 Behaviors indicating baby is attached to specific caregiver. (Source: (Ainsworth 1967)

Behavior	Example
Differential crying	Baby cries when held by stranger. Caregiver takes baby from stranger and baby stops crying
Differential smiling	Baby smiles frequently and readily at caregiver. Stranger smiles at baby. Baby smiles warily at stranger and turns away
Differential vocalization	Baby vocalizes more frequently and more readily during interactions with caregiver
Cries when caregiver leaves	Baby is playing contentedly on floor and seems oblivious to caregiver's presence. Caregiver leaves the room and baby begins to cry
Follows caregivers	Caregiver leaves the room and baby crawls after caregiver
Visual-motor orientation to caregivers	Baby is playing on floor. Caregiver walks across the room and baby watches her, turning to watch where caregiver is walking
Greeting responses	Caregiver comes into room and baby smiles, vocalizes, and reaches for caregiver
Scrambling	Climbing on mother. Playing with mother's hair or clothes
Burying face in caregiver's lap	Baby is standing by mother and stranger holds out toy for baby. Baby takes toy, turns, buries face in caregiver's lap
Approach through locomotion	Baby crawls towards caregiver
Kissing and hugging	Baby initiates hugs and kisses with caregiver. Baby molds to caregiver when caregiver hugs her
Use of the caregiver as a secure base for exploration	Dog enters room wagging its tail. Baby looks at parent and begins to crawl towards dog
Flight to caregiver as a haven of safety	Baby crawls near dog. Baby begins to cry, turns around, and crawls to caregiver
Clinging	Caregiver comforts frightened baby. Caregiver tries to put baby down on floor but baby continues to cling to caregiver

child. From the perspective of attachment theory, *not* becoming attached to one's primary caregivers or having only a "weak" attachment are highly unlikely. Failure to develop specific attachments to primary caregivers would be highly disadvantageous. Patterns of attachment are viewed as adaptive strategies that allow a child to maintain an attachment with less than optimal caregivers, albeit with some negative developmental consequences if the pattern is insecure.

Phases of Attachment Development

Ainsworth (1967; Ainsworth et al. 1978) and Bowlby (1969) identified four phases in the development of child-parent attachment. Over the first few months of development, children become increasingly active in maintaining the attachment relationship. By the time they have developed a clear-cut attachment towards the end of the first year, the infant has developed a pattern of relating to his primary caregivers based on his experiences with them. When they reach the fourth phase, around age 3 ½ or 4, the child-parent relationship has become a "goal-directed partnership" where true conflict and cooperation is possible. Descriptions of the phases of attachment development are summarized in Table 2.2.

Evaluating Quality of Attachment

In addition to looking for indicators of when a child became attached to a caregiver, Ainsworth used observations from her field studies to describe the quality of the attachment relationship. Ainsworth (1967) initially referred to this as the strength or security of the attachment relationship but in later writings exclusively used the term *security* (Ainsworth et al. 1978); "The obvious first impulse was to try to assess strength of attachment, but this ran up against a brick wall when one realized that this could not be achieved by the mere assessment of the strength or intensity of attachment behavior, for this is situational, and furthermore it is those who are anxiously attached who tend to have the strongest attachment behavior in the natural environment" (Ainsworth 1988).

Based on her extensive naturalistic observations of infant-mother interactions, Ainsworth et al. (1978) developed a standardized observational assessment known as the Strange Situation Procedure (SSP) to examine individual differences in the quality of infant-mother attachment. This procedure involves a series of situations designed to assess the balance between exploring the environment and seeking proximity to the attachment figure. The parent and child enter a novel playroom with attractive toys (designed to activate exploratory behavior). The baby is then confronted with a series of increasingly stressful situations designed to activate attachment behavior: the entrance of a stranger who first talks to the mother and then initiates interaction with the baby, an initial brief separation where the mother

Table 2.2 Phases of child-parent attachment. (Sources: (Ainsworth 1967; Ainsworth et al. 1978; Bowlby 1969))

Phase	Ainsworth label	Bowlby label	Approximate age	Description
1	Initial preattachment phase	Orientation and signals without discrimination of figure	Birth to 8–12 weeks	Uses signaling behaviors such as crying, smiling, and vocalizing to persuade people to approach. Uses rooting, sucking, and grasping to seek and maintain contact
2	Attachment-in-the-making	Orientation and signals directed towards one (or more) discriminated figures	12 weeks to about 6 months	Directs attachment behaviors (behaviors that promote proximity) towards specific individuals (primary caregivers). Attachment behaviors such as crying are more likely to be terminated by these attachment figures than other people. If preference for one or two preferred people over others is the criterion for attachment, the baby could be considered attached at this phase
3	Clear-cut attachment	Maintenance of proximity to a discriminated figure by means of locomotion as well as signals	Approximately 6 months to age 3 ½ or 4 (Onset delayed in infants who do not have limited number of primary caregivers)	Baby clearly discriminates between primary caregivers and other people. Baby actively seeks proximity with attachment figures through crawling and maintains contact through embracing and clinging. Greets primary caregivers when they return. Baby is active in exploring environment. Uses primary caregivers as secure base for exploration and safe haven when frightened. Baby learns to organize attachment behavior with reference to response of attachment figures (beginning of working model of attachment). Ainsworth views this onset of goal-corrected attachment behavior as the onset of attachment
4	Goal-corrected partnership	Goal-corrected partnership	Age 3 ½ or 4 through adulthood	Child is less egocentric and better able to see situations from caregiver's point of view. Language development facilitates development of more complex partnership. There is more recognition of conflicting agendas and child is better able to negotiate with parent and arrive at mutually acceptable compromises

leaves the child with the stranger, and a second brief separation where the child is left alone in the room. Each situation lasts 3 min. However, separations from the caregiver are curtailed early if the infant becomes distressed.

Based on observations of different aspects of the infant's or child's behavior in the SSP (e.g. proximity-seeking, contact-maintaining, avoidance, and resistance), the dyad is given a classification that summarizes the quality or pattern of attachment. In evaluating the security of the attachment relationship, the child's response to reunions with the mother following separations is especially important. Despite the complexity of the coding system, interrater reliability is good when the SSP is coded by well-trained observers (e.g. 80–90 % agreement; kappa = 0.69 to 0.72) (Cassidy et al. 2011; NICHD Early Child Care Research Network 1997). Information about training in coding the SSP is available at the Attachment Training web site: http://attachment-training.com/at/. The SSP is considered the "gold standard" for assessing the quality of infant-parent attachment due to the extensive research supporting its relationship to in-home observations and longitudinal outcomes (Zeanah et al. 2011).

The three patterns of attachment originally identified by Ainsworth et al. (1978) are now referred to as organized patterns of attachment. When Ainsworth first described these different patterns of attachment, she assigned a letter to each type, a shorthand that has stuck over the years. Securely attached infants and young children (B) exhibit a balance between proximity-seeking and exploration. They directly communicate distress in situations that provoke uncertainty or fear, seek proximity to their mother when distressed, are soothed by their mother, and return to exploration. In the other two organized patterns of attachment, the baby or young child is primarily focused on seeking and maintaining proximity to the primary caregiver (insecure-ambivalent/resistant) (C) or is primarily focused on exploring the environment (insecure-avoidant) (A) rather than exhibiting a balance between proximity-seeking and exploration. In the first four samples where Ainsworth used this classification system (N = 106), 66 % of dyads exhibited a secure attachment (B), 22 % exhibited an avoidant attachment (A), and 12 % exhibited an ambivalent/resistant attachment (C) (Ainsworth et al. 1978).

The classification of disorganized attachment (D) was developed by Main and Solomon (1990) after reviewing videotapes of dyads that were difficult to "fit" into Ainsworth's organized attachment classifications. The infants in these dyads exhibit a variety of conflict behaviors in stressful situations when they are in the presence of their caregiver. These conflict behaviors are not consistent with the organized patterns identified by Ainsworth and came to be understood as a breakdown in the infant's ability to effectively use the mother for emotional regulation under stressful circumstances (Main and Solomon 1990; van Ijzendoorn et al. 1999). Breakdowns sufficient to classify a dyad as disorganized can range from brief interruptions in an otherwise organized pattern of attachment to global disorganization.

The majority of infant-mother dyads classified as disorganized are given a secondary, best-fitting Ainsworth et al. (1978) classification. For example, an infant classified as disorganized/secure[2] (D/B) might exhibit an overall pattern of going to their parent for comfort when distressed but exhibit conflict behaviors in the context of comfort-seeking (e.g. briefly freezing or engaging in stereotypies such as hair twisting or rocking on the approach to the parent or turning around and backing toward the parent for comfort). In the relatively rare circumstance where the dyad exhibits global disorganization and a secondary classification cannot be determined, the dyad is classified as disorganized/cannot classify.

The SSP and coding system has been modified for use with young children (ages 2 through 6) (Cassidy et al. 1992) and 6-year-olds (Main and Cassidy 1985). There is a growing body of literature on the modified SSP for preschool-aged children, making it the best-validated assessment of attachment security for young children (Greenberg et al. 1991; Moss et al. 2004; Speltz et al. 1990, 1995, 1999). Like the infant SSP, the preschool adaptation uses brief separations from the caregiver. In early studies, the infant procedure was followed but separations were lengthened. In later studies, there continue to be longer separations than used for infants (5 min vs. 3 min) but a stranger is not used. The modified SSP for pre-schoolers used in current studies is as follows: The parent and child enter a playroom for 5 min. The parent then leaves for 5 min, returns for 5 min, leaves a second time for 5 min, and returns a second time for 5 min (Moss et al. 2004, 2011). The procedure for 6-year-olds uses a 1 h separation where the child is with a stranger and only one reunion (Main and Cassidy 1985).

When evaluating quality of attachment in infants and young children, it is important to recognize the major developmental shifts that occur between infancy and early childhood. For example, while securely attached infants often cry during the 3 min SSP separations, securely attached pre-schoolers rarely cry during 5 min separations.

Striking developmental shifts from infancy to school-age are seen in longitudinal studies of infants with a disorganized attachment relationship (Hesse and Main 2000). Many of the school-aged children who display the conflict behaviors and anxiety indicative of disorganized attachment as infants display a controlling pattern of interacting with their parent as 6-year-olds. It is as though they have resolved their conflict and anxiety by taking charge of the relationship. Details of the patterns of attachment in infants and pre-schoolers are presented in Table 2.3.

Positive Parenting Behaviors—Attachment Perspective

The parenting behavior identified in Ainsworth's research as central to the development of secure attachment is sensitive responsiveness, i.e. the parent's prompt, consistent, and appropriate response to the baby's attachment signals (Ainsworth

[2] Dyads with a disorganized/secure attachment classification are considered insecurely attached, a confusing aspect of attachment nomenclature that has led Lyons-Ruth and Spielman (2004) to refer to this group as disorganized-approach.

Table 2.3 Characteristics of attachment patterns in infant and preschool child-caregiver dyads. (Sources: (Ainsworth et al. 1978; Cassidy and Marvin 1992; Main and Solomon 1990))

Pattern	Infant-parent	Preschooler-parent
Secure (B)	The baby may be distressed during separations from caregiver. If she is distressed, she seeks contact with the parent during the reunions and is easily soothed by the parent. The baby actively seeks interaction with parent after separation with little resistance or avoidance. The baby clearly acknowledges parent's return following separations with smile, cry, or approach	Child is interested in interacting with the parent. Child rarely shows extensive crying during separation but may exhibit muted exploration or search for parent. Child may exhibit no distress during separation—continuing to play until parent returns. Child displays relaxed pleasure at parent's return and interaction picks up where it left off prior to separation
Ambivalent/ Resistant (C)	The baby is distressed during separations. During the reunions, the baby both resists and seeks contact with the caregiver	Child is very focused on interacting with the parent and displays little exploratory behavior. May be highly distressed during separation. During the reunions, both seeks and resists contact. May tantrum, whine, or hit the parent
Avoidant (A)	The baby is not distressed during separation when the stranger is present. Ignores parent's return, often by feigning interest in toys. Avoids proximity to mother during reunion	Child is focused on exploration and displays little interest in interactions which indicate a special relationship with parent. During the reunions, child may avoid parent or may engage in interactions that appear civil but formal
[a]Disorganized/Controlling (D)	When caregiver is present, child displays (1) sequential display of contradictory behavior patterns, (2) simultaneous display of contradictory behavior patterns, (3) undirected, misdirected, incomplete, and interrupted movements and expressions, (4) stereotypies, asymmetrical movements, mistimed movements, and anomalous postures, (5) freezing, stilling, and slowed movements and expressions, (6) direct indices of apprehension regarding the parent, or (7) direct indices of disorganization or disorientation	Disorganized: When caregiver is present, child displays (1) disordering of expected sequence of behavior, (2) incomplete or undirected movements, (3) confusion or apprehension, dazed or disoriented expression, or depressed affect. Disorganized/Controlling: During reunion, child takes control of the interaction

[a]A best-fitting secondary pattern is also assigned—e.g. D/A

et al. 1978). As shown in Table 2.1, attachment signals include both affectively positive signals (e.g. smiling, reaching, following) and affectively negative signals (e.g. crying). Subsequent research suggests sensitive responsiveness to infant distress is especially important in the development of a secure infant-parent attachment (Del Carmen et al. 1993; van den Boom 1988, 1989, 1994). However, it is important to note the distinction between sensitive responsiveness and responsiveness. Sensitive responsiveness involves both knowing when to respond to a baby and when to let the baby utilize their emerging capacities for self-regulation (Beebe et al. 2010; van IJzendoorn and Hubbard 2000). Research indicates a curvilinear relationship between responsiveness and secure attachment suggesting sensitive responsiveness involves the "just right" amount of responsiveness - neither too much nor too little (Beebe et al. 2010).

The parenting behavior with the strongest empirical support for its association with attachment is sensitive responsiveness. However, this parenting behavior explains only a portion of the variance in security of attachment. Table 2.4 summarizes some of the other parenting behaviors associated with the development of secure attachment.

Insecure attachment is clearly a risk factor for disruptive behavior; a meta-analysis of 69 studies examining the association of attachment and externalizing behavior problems found a statistically significant association ($d=0.31$) (Fearon et al. 2010). Disorganized attachment had a stronger association with externalizing behavior problems ($d=0.34$) than avoidance ($d=0.12$) or resistance ($d=0.11$).

Research on Attachment Theory-Based Interventions

Numerous interventions targeting infants/young children and their parents cite attachment theory as a theoretical foundation and indicate their intervention improves attachment (Bakermans-Kranenburg et al. 2003, 2005; Bernard et al. 2012; Cassidy et al. 2011; Chaffin et al. 2011; Cohen et al. 1999; Dozier et al. 2002, 2007; Eyberg 2005; Hoffman et al. 2006; Ijzendoorn 1995; Moss et al. 2011; Sanders 2010; van den Boom 1988, 1989, 1994). This review focuses on interventions with outcome studies utilizing research-based observational assessments of attachment security (SSP or Modified SSP for Preschoolers).

Watch, Wait, and Wonder (WWW), Infant-Parent/Child-Parent Psychotherapy (CPP), and Circle of Security (COS) are described below and outcome studies of these interventions are summarized in Table 2.5. Watch, Wait, and Wonder (WWW) is the only attachment-based intervention demonstrated to ameliorate insecure attachment among infants and toddlers referred for mental health concerns (Cohen et al. 1999). WWW is a dyadic, child-led approach based on attachment theory and object relations theory (specifically, Winnicott and Bion's concepts of the holding environment and projective identification). During the first half of the session (20–30 min), the mother is encouraged to get down on the floor with her infant or child and follow his lead. The mother is told if her child initiates an interaction with her

Table 2.4 Parenting behaviors associated with secure attachment. (Sources: (Ainsworth 1967; Ainsworth et al. 1978; Beebe et al. 2010; Bernier et al. 2014; Britner et al. 2005; De Wolff and Van Ijzendoorn 1997))

Behavior	Definition	Examples
Sensitive responsiveness	Parent exhibits prompt, consistent, and appropriate responses to infant's attachment signals	Parent picks up fussing child and pats her back. Parent picks up child who is smiling and reaching for her
Support for exploration	Parent provides a secure base for exploration of the environment by attending to child's exploration and scaffolding problem-solving on difficult tasks	Child crawls away from parent to investigate toys, picks up block, turns, and shows it to parent. Parent smiles encouragingly and says "Did you find a block?" Child is walking around room by holding on to furniture and gets to a gap. Parent holds out fingers to support child until he reaches the next piece of furniture
Synchronous interaction	Parent-child interactions appear reciprocal and mutually rewarding. Parent is neither intrusive nor unresponsive. Interactions are characterized by turn-taking. This has been described as "serve and return"	Baby smiles at mother, babbles, and quiets. Parent says "Are you telling me about your day?" Baby babbles again
Attunement	Parent facial expressions and behaviors indicating parent is in tune with child's inner state	Baby fusses. Parent exhibits sympathetic facial expression as he picks up baby. Baby crawls quickly towards toys. Parent exhibits excited facial expression as she says animatedly "You are excited to play, aren't you?"
Delight in child	Positive affect towards child or child's activities	Child is sitting on floor examining his hands. Parent looks at child and beams
Positive physical contact	Positive physical contact between parent and child initiated by either parent or child. Positive physical contact when the child is distressed is especially important to the development of a secure attachment	Child fusses and parent picks him up and rubs his back. Child leans against parent's knee and parent leans down and hugs child

Table 2.5 Attachment-based intervention studies

Population	Model	Rate of secure attachment	Drop-out rate	Reference
Infants and toddlers referred for mental health services (Canada) *N*=66	Watch, Wait, and Wonder (WWW): Child-Parent Psychotherapy (CPP)	Pre WWW: 18% Post WWW: 26% Pre CPP: 28% Post CPP: 12%	9%	Cohen et al. 1999
Infants in maltreating families (United States) *N*=137	Child-Parent Psychotherapy (CPP) Nurse-Family Partnership (NFP) Community Services (CS)	Pre CPP: 3% Post CPP: 61% Pre NFP: 0% Post NFP: 54% Pre CS: 0% Post CS: 2%	CPP: 12% NFP: 8% CS: 33%	Cicchetti et al. 2006
Toddlers of mothers with postpartum major depressive disorder (United States) N=130	Child-Parent Psychotherapy (CPP) Treatment as Usual (TAU)	Pre CPP: 17% Post CPP: 67% Pre TAU: 22% Post TAU: 17%	CPP: 30% TAU: 13%	Toth et al. 2006
At-risk Head Start and Early Head Start preschoolers (United States) *N*=65	Circle of security (COS): Pre: 20% Post: 54%	Pre COS: 20% Post COS: 54%	0	Hoffman et al. 2006
First born, irritable, economically stressed infants (United States) *N*=220	Circle of security-Home visiting—4 intervention (COS-HV4) Control (Con)	COS-HV4: 60% Con: 50%	COS-HV4: 5% Con: 4%	Cassidy et al. 2011

she should respond, keeping her child's agenda in mind and not introducing her own agenda. She is told that if she is not sure what to do, she should remember "Watch, Wait, and Wonder." In the second half of the session (20–30 min), the therapist asks the mother about her observations of the child, her experience of doing child-led play, and any difficulties she had doing child-led play.

Infant-Parent Psychotherapy/Child-Parent Psychotherapy (CPP) is an intervention developed by Selma Fraiberg (CPP became the inclusive title when Infant-Parent Psychotherapy was extended to toddlers and preschool-aged children) (Fraiberg 1980; Fraiberg et al. 1975; Lieberman and Van Horn 2008). Fraiberg, who was trained as a social worker and psychoanalyst, developed CPP as a home visiting model focused on improving infant-parent interactions. The premise of this approach is disturbances in child-parent relationships result from the parent's psychological conflicts being expressed through the parent's attitudes and behaviors toward the infant and the best way to address these disturbances is working directly with the child-parent dyad. The primary modality is joint child-parent sessions where spontaneous child-parent interactions are used to support the child's positive development and address parental conflicts that may be a barrier to healthy development. Some of the strategies therapists use include "speaking for the baby" to help the parent recognize the meaning of the child's behavior, developmental guidance, crisis intervention, and helping the parent recognize how exposure to traumatic events has impacted their interactions. A core theoretical tenet of CPP is that when the parent is able to remember the affect associated with a painful event they are able to become protective of their child rather than acting out past traumas in their interactions with their child. In the outcome studies reported in Table 2.5, CPP lasted 5–12 months (number of sessions ranged from 15–45). As shown in Table 2.5, CPP leads to significant increases in security of attachment in dyads with maltreating parents (Cicchetti et al. 2006) and mothers with Postpartum Major Depression (Toth et al. 2006). However, in the only study examining changes in attachment security in a clinically-referred population, families receiving CPP exhibited a decrease in secure attachment following treatment (Cohen et al. 1999).

Circle of Security protocols (Cassidy et al. 2007, 2011; Cooper et al. 2005; Hoffman et al. 2006) use education about secure attachment to target parents' sensitive responsiveness to their child's attachment signals. In the 20-week COS group intervention protocol, at-risk parents are videotaped with their child during a modified SSP for preschoolers, reading a book together, and toy clean-up (Cooper et al. 2005; Hoffman et al. 2006; Powell et al. 2014). An individualized treatment plan targeting the most problematic aspect of the child-parent relationship is used to select video segments that will increase her capacity to reflect on her caregiving and show her examples where she is demonstrating underutilized capacities. As shown in Table 2.5, this COS protocol is associated with significant increases in secure attachment. The Circle of Security-Home Visiting-4 Intervention (COS-HV4) protocol developed for mothers of irritable babies consists of four home visits designed to help mothers attend to both attachment and exploratory behaviors. The intervention focuses on helping mothers enhance their observations of their infant, select and implement sensitive responses, and help the mother reflect on how her cognitive and reflective responses may influence her behavior. As shown in Table 2.5, mothers participating in the COS-HV4 intervention were only slightly more likely to have a secure attachment relationship with their baby (differences were not statistically significant) (Cassidy et al. 2011). However, the intervention did increase security of attachment for dyads with highly irritable babies.

Research on Attachment Theory-Based Parent Coaching

Results of attachment-based interventions utilizing parent coaching are described below and summarized in Table 2.6. These approaches utilize in vivo coaching while parents are interacting with their child, parent video feedback using videos of the parent interacting with their child, or a combination of these coaching approaches. The emphasis is on encouraging behaviors that promote secure attachment and gently prompting parents to change parenting behaviors that undermine attachment security.

The skills-based coaching intervention for irritable babies developed by Dymph van den Boom is a brief (3 session) home visiting intervention that uses detailed coding of mother-infant interactions to guide parent coaching (van den Boom 1988, 1989, 1994). Coding of the infant's attachment signals and the mother's response to the signals are used to guide the interventionist's coaching during the home visit. For example, if the mother is intrusive and overstimulating, the home visitor has the mother sit back and describe what the infant is doing. If the infant cries during the home visit, the interventionist prompts the mother to pick up the baby and focuses on the mother's effectiveness at soothing the baby and the importance of responding to infant crying. As shown in Table 2.6, this brief, skills-based intervention was highly effective at increasing security of attachment.

Relationship Intervention Program, a brief (8 session) home-visiting intervention utilizes video feedback of joint child-parent play to improve parental sensitive responsiveness in families with a confirmed report of child maltreatment (physical abuse, neglect, or sexual abuse) of a young child (aged 1–6) (Moss et al. 2011). Video feedback is used to focus on positive parent-child sequences and reinforce the parent's sensitive responsiveness to the child's attachment signals. As shown in Table 2.6, the majority of dyads participating in the Relationship Intervention Program become securely attached following the intervention while there is relatively little change in the group receiving community services.

Video-feedback Intervention to Promote Positive Parenting (VIPP) protocols videotape children interacting with their parents and view these videos with parents to enhance sensitive responsiveness (Bakermans-Kranenburg et al. 1998, 2008a, 2008b; Juffer et al. 2005) During the joint viewing of the videos, the interventionist comments on moments where the mother is sensitively responsive to the baby's attachment signals. When viewing interactions where the mother missed the infant's attachment cues, the provider "speaks for the baby" to help increase the caregiver's sensitive responsiveness. As shown in Table 2.6, the brief (3 session) VIPP protocol developed for caregivers of adopted infants failed to lead to increased secure attachment in this group where the rate of secure attachment was already quite high (75 % in the control group) (Juffer et al. 2005). However, VIPP did decrease disorganized attachment (see Chap. 8).

Attachment and Biobehavioral Catch-up (ABC) is a brief (10 session) intervention focusing on increasing sensitive, nurturing care and decreasing frightening behavior (Bernard et al. 2012; Dozier et al. 2002, 2008). ABC uses both video feedback and in the moment coaching to target increases in sensitive responsiveness and decreases in frightening behavior.

Internal Working Models of Attachment in Adults

An important development in the study of attachment was the development of methodology for studying adult's internal working models of attachment. Bowlby proposed the quality of early attachment relationships impacts our perceptions and representations of later relationships (Bowlby 1969). The Adult Attachment Interview (AAI) was developed by Mary Main and Ruth Goldwyn to assess this "move to the level of representation" in adolescents and adults (Main and Goldwyn 1998). The AAI is an hour long interview where individuals are asked about their relationships with their parents and childhood experiences. This interview is transcribed verbatim and coded to provide an assessment of working model of attachment or what they came to call "state of mind". Coders first complete inferred-experience scales reflecting their impression of individual's experiences with caregivers during childhood. Main and Goldwyn's (1998) critical insight was that determination of attachment state of mind is based on how individuals tell the stories of their childhoods (i.e. process) rather than the content of the stories. That is, parents who describe significant setbacks, harsh parenting, and even abuse have securely attached relationships with their children when they tell these stories in a fresh, genuine, and

Table 2.6 Attachment-based parent coaching

Population	Model	Rate of secure attachment	Drop-out rate	Reference
First born, irritable, low socioeconomic infants (Netherlands) *N*=100 at 12 mos; 82 at 18 mos	Skill-based intervention (SBI Control (Con)	12 mos Post SBI: 62% Post Con.: 22% 18 mos Post SBI: 72% Post Con.: 26%	0%	van den Boom 1994
Adopted infants (Netherlands) *N*=98	Video-feedback Intervention to Promote Positive Parenting (VIPP) Control (Con)	Post VIPP: 72% Post Con: 75%	0%	Juffer et al. 2005
Maltreated infants and preschool-aged children (Canada) *N*=66	Relationship Intervention Program (RIP) Community Services (CS)	Pre RIP: 25% Post RIP: 66% Pre CS: 22% Post CS: 28%	RIP: 7% CS: 15%	Moss et al. 2011
Infants and toddlers at risk for maltreatment (United States) N=120 children/113 parents	Attachment and biobehavioral catch-up (ABC) Developmental education for families (DEF)	Post ABC: 52% Post DEF: 33%	0%	Bernard et al. 2012

forgiving manner. As with the SSP, interrater reliability is good for well-trained coders (92–95 % agreement; kappa = 0.84 to 0.89) (Booth-LaForce and Roisman 2014; Caspers et al. 2007). Information about training in coding the AAI is available at the Attachment Training web site: http://attachment-training.com/at/.

A meta-analysis of the predictive validity of the AAI indicates a significant association between secure/autonomous parental state of mind and infant-parent attachment security (effect size = 1.06; percent agreement = 75 %) (Van Ijzendoorn 1995). The concordance between parental AAI and infant attachment is even higher than the concordance between behavioral observations of sensitive responsiveness and attachment leading van Ijzendoorn (1995) to describe a "transmission gap" between state of mind and security of attachment. These results indicate paying attention to factors not observed during observations of parents such as how parents talk about their own childhoods and therapists' emotional reactions to the parent may provide information that supplements information obtained from observations of parent-child interactions. Characteristics of secure and insecure states of mind are summarized in Table 2.7. Infant/child patterns of attachment corresponding to adult attachment states of mind and rates in community samples are summarized in Table 2.8.

Table 2.7 Summary of adult attachment state of mind (based on Adult Attachment Interview (AAI). (Sources: (Main and Goldwyn 1998; Steele and Steele 2008))

Secure/Autonomous (F)	Values attachment relationships and experiences. Generalized descriptions of relationships with parents (semantic level) are supported by specific memories. Adult either supports descriptions of parents as loving during childhood (continuous secure) or reflects on parents' lack of loving behavior without angry preoccupation or idealization (earned secure)
Preoccupied with attachment figures and experiences (E)	Preoccupied with early attachment experiences. Vacillates between positive and negative evaluations of parents. Extensive discussion of feelings, experiences, and relationships that is confused and lacks coherence
Dismissing of attachment (Ds)	Dismisses the importance of early attachment relationships by failing to recognize negative early experiences and/or negative effects of difficult early experiences. Generalized descriptions of relationships with parents (semantic level) are not supported by specific memories, attachment figures are devalued, or adult reports he was not affected by early experiences or negative experiences made him stronger
Unresolved (disorganized/disoriented) with respect to experiences of loss or abuse by attachment figure (Ud)	Lapses in the monitoring of reasoning or discourse when discussing a loss (e.g. speaking of deceased as though they are still alive, prolonged silences) or abuse (e.g. becomes incoherent when discussing abuse, alternates report of abuse with denial of abuse)

Table 2.8 Rates of attachment patterns and corresponding states of mind in community samples. (Sources: (Ainsworth et al. 1978; Bakermans-Kranenburg and van Ijzendoorn 2009; Booth-LaForce & Roisman, 2014; Caspers et al., 2007; Greenberg et al. 1991; Main and Goldwyn 1998; Moss et al. 2004; Speltz et al. 1990, 1999, Troutman et al. 2010; van Ijzendoorn et al. 1999))

Infant-parent Strange Situation Procedure (SSP)	Preschool child-parent modified Strange situation procedure (SSP)	Adult state of mind Adult Attachment Interview (AAI)
Secure (B) 55–62%	Secure (B) 57–78%	Secure/Autonomous (F) 48–59%
Ambivalent/Resistant (C) 4–12%	Ambivalent/Resistant (C) 4–10%	Preoccupied (E) 3–10%
Avoidant (A) 7–15%	Avoidant (A) 7–15%	Dismissing (Ds) 15–35%
[a]Disorganized (D) 15%	*Disorganized (D)/ Controlling-Disorganized (D) 11–15%	[a]Unresolved/Disorganized (Ud) 3–18%

[a]A best-fitting secondary pattern is also assigned—e.g. D/A or Ud/E

Research on Adult Attachment State of Mind

In addition to predicting security of infant-parent attachment, research on the AAI indicates attachment states of mind are associated with parenting behaviors and adults' physiological responses to infant attachment signals (Riem et al. 2012). Attachment state of mind is also associated with willingness to seek psychological treatment, types of psychological services the individual willingly engages in, and providers' attitudes toward the individual (Korfmacher et al. 1997; Riem et al. 2012). More information about these studies and the clinical implications of this research for parent coaching is provided in Chaps. 5, 6, 7, and 8.

Adult Attachment Intervention Studies

In a small study of patients with child abuse-related Posttraumatic Stress Disorder who received either Prolonged Exposure (PE) and Skills Training in Affective and Emotional Regulation (STAIR) there was a significant increase in secure/autonomous state of mind (Stovall-McClough and Cloitre 2003). In a study of patients with Borderline Personality Disorder, Transference-Focused Psychotherapy (TFP), a psychodynamic intervention focusing on modifying representations of self and others through interpretation of the transference relationship, led to a significant increase in secure/autonomous state of mind while Dialectical Behavior Therapy (DBT) and Supportive Psychotherapy (SPT) were not associated with changes in state of mind (Levy et al. 2006). A year long home visiting and group parenting intervention program focused on improving maternal sensitivity and secure attachment (Steps Toward Effective, Enjoyable Parenting (STEEP) found similar rates of secure/autonomous

Table 2.9 Rates of secure/autonomous state of mind in intervention studies

Population	Model	Rate of secure/ autonomous state of mind	Reference
First time, low income mothers (United States) $N=154$	Steps toward effective, enjoyable parenting (STEEP) control (Con)	Post STEEP: 47 % Post Con: 57 %	Erickson et al. 1992
Patients receiving psychotherapy for borderline personality disorder (United States) $N=90$	Transference-focused psychotherapy (TFP) Dialectical behavior therapy (DBT) Supportive psychotherapy (SPT)	Pre TFP: 5 % Post TFP: 32 % Pre DBT: 6 % Post DBT: 6 % Pre SPT: 5 % Post SPT: 5 %	Levy et al. 2006
Patients receiving psychotherapy for child abuse-related posttraumatic stress disorder (United States) $N=18$	Prolonged exposure (PE) or skills training in affective and interpersonal regulation (STAIR)	Pre PE or STAIR: 11 % Post PE or STAIR: 50 %	Stovall-McClough and Cloitre 2003

state of mind in the intervention and control group following the intervention (Korfmacher et al. 1997). Results of these studies are summarized in Table 2.9.

Conclusions

Research on interventions based on attachment theory indicate interventions that build on attachment theory research, especially regarding the role of sensitive responsiveness, are associated with improvements in the quality of infant-parent and child-parent attachment. This outcomes research provides clear evidence it is possible to promote secure attachment, prevent insecure attachment, and ameliorate insecure attachment, even in highly stressed populations such as maltreating parents.

Research on adult attachment state of mind indicates it is possible for adults to develop a more secure state of mind in psychotherapy, providing hope that prevention work can begin even before children are born. The shortcoming of current knowledge about addressing insecure attachment is the lack of evidence-based attachment interventions for young children exhibiting clinically significant levels of disruptive behavior.

References

Ainsworth, M. (1967). *Infancy in Uganda*. Baltimore: Johns Hopkins.

Ainsworth, M., Blehar, M., Waters, E., & Wall, S. (1978). *Patterns of attachment: A psychological study of the strange situation*. Hillsdale: Erlbaum.

Ainsworth, M. (1988). On security. http://www.psychology.sunysb.edu/attachment/pdf/mda_security.pdf. Accessed 6 July 2014.

Bakermans-Kranenburg, M., & van Ijzendoorn, M. (2009). The first 10,000 adult attachment interviews: Distributions of adult attachment representations in clinical and non-clinical groups. *Attachment & Human Development, 11*(3), 223–263.

Bakermans-Kranenburg, M. J., Juffer, F., & van Ijzendoorn, M. H. (1998). Interventions with video feedback and attachment discussions: Does type of maternal insecurity make a difference? *Infant Mental Health Journal, 19*(2), 202–219.

Bakermans-Kranenburg, M. J., van Ijzendoorn, M. H., & Juffer, F. (2003). Less is more: Meta-analyses of sensitivity and attachment interventions in early childhood. *Psychological Bulletin, 129*(2), 195–215.

Bakermans-Kranenburg, M. J., Van Ijzendoorn, M. H., & Juffer, F. (2005). Disorganized infant attachment and preventive interventions: A review and meta-analysis. *Infant Mental Health Journal, 26*(3), 191–216.

Bakermans-Kranenburg, M., Breddels-van Baardewijk, P., Juffer, F., Klein Velderman, M., & Van IJzendoorn, M. (2008a). Insecure mothers with temperamentally reactive infants: A chance for intervention. In F. Juffer, M. Bakermans-Kranenburg, & M. van Ijzendoorn (Eds.), *Promoting positive parenting: An attachment-based intervention* (pp. 75–90). New York: Lawrence Erlbaum Associates.

Bakermans-Kranenburg, M., van IJzendoorn, M., Pijlman, F., Mesman, J., & Juffer, F. (2008b). Experimental evidence for differential susceptibility: Dopamine D4 receptor polymorphism (DRD4 VNTR) moderates intervention effects on toddlers' externalizing behavior in a randomized controlled trial. *Developmental Psychology, 44*(1), 293–300.

Beebe, B., Jaffe, J., Markese, S., Buck, K., Chen, H., Cohen, P., Bahrick, L., Andrews, H., & Feldstein, S. (2010). The origins of 12-month attachment: A microanalysis of 4-month mother-infant interaction. *Attachment & Human Development, 12*(1), 3–141.

Bernard, K., Dozier, M., Bick, J., Lewis-Morrarty, E., Lindhiem, O., & Carlson, E. (2012). Enhancing attachment organization among maltreated children: Results of a randomized clinical trial. *Child Development, 83*(2), 623–636.

Bernier, A., Matte-Gagne, C., Belanger, M., & Whipple, N. (2014). Taking stock of two decades of attachment transmission gap: Broadening the assessment of maternal behavior. *Child Development, 85* (5), 1852–1865.

Booth-LaForce, C., & Roisman, G. (2014). The adult attachment interview: Psychometrics, stability and change from infancy, and develpmental origins. *Monographs of the Society for Research in Child Development, 79*(3), 1–185.

Bowlby, J. (1969). *Attachment and loss. Vol 1: Attachment*. New York: Basic Books.

Britner, P., Marvin, R., & Pianta, R. (2005). Development and preliminary validation of the caregiving behavior system: Association with child attachment classification in the preschool strange situation. *Attachment & Human Development, 7,* 83–102.

Caspers, K., Yucuis, R., Troutman, B., Arndt, S., & Langbehn, D. (2007). A sibling adoption study of adult attachment: The influence of shared environment on attachment state of mind. *Attachment & Human Development, 9*(4), 375–391.

Cassidy, J., & Marvin, R. (1992). *Attachment organization in three and four year olds: Procedures and coding manual*. University of Virginia.

Cassidy, J., Marvin, R., & the MacArthur Working Group on Attachment. (1992). *Attachment organization in preschool children: Procedures and coding guidelines* (4th ed.). University of Virginia. Charlottesville.

Cassidy, J., Ziv, Y., Cooper, G., Hoffman, K., Powell, B., & Karfgin, A. (2007). *Enhancing attachment security in the infants of women in a jail-diversion program*. Paper presented at the Biennial meeting of the Social for Research in Child Development, Boston.

Cassidy, J., Woodhouse, S., Sherman, L., Stupica, B., & Lejuez, C. W. (2011). Enhancing infant attachment security: An examination of treatment efficacy and differential susceptibility. *Development and Psychopathology, 23,* 131–148.

Chaffin, M., Funderburk, B., Bard, D., Valle, L., & Gurwitch, R. (2011). A combined motivation and parent-child interaction therapy package reduces child welfare recidivism in a randomized dismantling field trial. *Journal of Consulting and Clinical Psychology, 79*(1), 84–95.

Cicchetti, D., Rogosch, F., & Toth, S. (2006). Fostering secure attachment in infants in maltreating families through preventive interventions. *Development and Psychopathology, 18,* 623–649.

Cohen, N., Muir, E., Lojkasek, M., Muir, R., Parker, C., Barwick, M., & Brown, M. (1999). Watch, wait and wonder: Testing the effectiveness of a new approahc to mother-infant psychotherapy. *Infant Mental Health Journal, 20,* 429–451.

Cooper, G., Hoffman, K., Powell, B., & Marvin, R. (2005). The Circle of Security Intervention: Differential diagnosis and differential treatment. In L. Berlin, Y. Ziv, L. Amaya-Jackson, & M. Greenberg (Eds.), *Enhancing early attachments: Theory, research, intervention, and policy* (pp. 127–151). New York: Guilford.

De Wolff, M., & Van Ijzendoorn, M. (1997). Sensitivity and attachment: A meta-analysis on parental antecedents of infant attachment. *Child Development, 68*(4), 571–591.

Del Carmen, R., Pedersen, F., Huffman, L., & Bryan, Y. (1993). Dyadic distress management predicts subsequent security of attachment. *Infant Behavior and Development, 16,* 131–147.

Dozier, M., Higley, E., Albus, K., & Nutter, A. (2002). Intervening with foster infants' caregivers: Targeting three critical needs. *Infant Mental Health Journal, 23*(5), 541–554.

Dozier, M., Peloso, E., Zirkel, S., & Lindheim, O. (2007). *Intervention effects on foster infants'attachment to new caregivers.* Paper presented at the Society for Research in Child Development, Boston.

Dozier, M., Peloso, E., Lewis, E., Laurenceau, J., & Levine, S. (2008). Effects of an attachment-based intervention on the cortisol production of infants and toddlers in foster care. *Development and Psychopathology, 20,* 845–859.

Erickson, M., Korfmacher, J., & Egeland, B. (1992). Attachments past and present: Implications for therapeutic intervention with mother-infant dyads. *Development and Psychopathology, 4,* 495–507.

Eyberg, S. (2005). Parent-child interaction therapy: Basic coaching guidelines. Retrieved August 13, 2013, from University of Florida PCIT website: pcit.phhp.ufl.edu/.../web%20Coaching%20in%20PCIT%20May%202006.ppt.

Fearon, R., Bakermans-Kranenburg, M., van Ijzendoorn, M., Lapsley, A., & Roisman, G. (2010). The significance of insecure attachment and disorganization in the development of children's externalizing behavior: A meta-analytic study. *Child Development, 81*(2), 435–456.

Fraiberg, S. (1980). *Clinical studies in infant mental health: The first year of life.* New York: Basic Books.

Fraiberg, S., Adelson, E., & Shapiro, V. (1975). Ghosts in the nursery: A psychoanalytic approach to impaired infant-mother relationships. *Journal of the American Academy of Child Psychiatry, 14,* 387–421.

Greenberg, M., Speltz, M., DeKlyen, M., & Endriga, M. (1991). Attachment security in preschoolers with and without externalizing behavior problems: A replication. *Development and Psychopathology, 3,* 413–430.

Hesse, E., & Main, M. (2000). Disorganized infant, child, and adult attachment: Collapse in behavioral and attentional strategies. *Journal of the American Psychoanalytic Association,* 48(4), 1097–1127.

Hoffman, K., Marvin, R., Cooper, G., & Powell, B. (2006). Changing toddlers' and preschoolers' attachment classifications: The circle of security intervention. *Journal of Consulting and Clinical Psychology, 74,* 1017–1026.

Ijzendoorn, M. v. (1995). Breaking the intergenerational cycle of insecure attachment: A review of the effects of attachment-based interventions on maternal sensitivity and infant security. *Journal of Child Psychology and Psychiatry, 36,* 225–248.

Juffer, F., Bakermans-Kranenburg, M. J., & van Ijzendoorn, M. H. (2005). The importance of parenting in the development of disorganized attachment: Evidence from a preventive intervention study in adoptive families. *Journal of Child Psychology and Psychiatry, 46*(3), 263–274.

Korfmacher, J., Adam, E., Ogawa, J., & Egeland, B. (1997). Adult attachment: Implications for the therapeutic process in a home visitation intervention *Applied Developmental Science, 1*(1), 43–52.

Levy, K., Meehan, K., Kelly, K., Reynoso, J., Weber, M., Clarkin, J., & Kernberg, O. (2006). Change in attachment patterns and reflective function in a randomized control trial of transference-focused psychotherapy for borderline personality disorder. *Journal of Consulting and Clinical Psychology, 74*(6), 1027–1040.

Lieberman, A. F., & Van Horn, P. (2008). *Psychotherapy with infants and young children: Repairing the effects of stress and trauma on early attachment*. New York: Guilford.

Lyons-Ruth, K., & Spielman, E. (2004). Disorganized infant attachment strategies and helpless-fearful profiles of parenting: Integrating attachment research with clinical intervention. *Infant Mental Health Journal, 25*(4), 318–335.

Main, M., & Cassidy, J. (1985). Assessments of child-parent attachment at six years of age. Unpublished manuscript.

Main, M., & Goldwyn, R. (1998). *Adult attachment scoring and classification system*. Berkeley: University of California.

Main, M., & Solomon, J. (1990). Procedures for identifying infants as disorganized/disoriented during the Ainsworth Strange situation. In M. Greenberg, D. Cicchetti, & E. Cummings (Eds.), *Attachment in the preschool years: Theory, research, and intervention*. Chicago: The University of Chicago Press.

Moss, E., Cyr, C., & Dubois-Comtois, K. (2004). Attachment at early school age and developmental risk: Examining family contexts and behavior problems of controlling-caregiving, controlling-punitive, and behaviorally disorganized children. *Developmental Psychology, 40*(4), 519–532.

Moss, E., Dubois-Comtois, K., Cyr, C., St-Laurent, D., & Bernier, A. (2011). Efficacy of a home-visiting intervention aimed at improving maternal sensitivity, child attachment, and behavioral outcomes for maltreated children: A randomized control trial. *Development and Psychopathology, 23,* 195–210.

NICHD Early Child Care Research Network. (1997). The effects of infant child care on infant-mother attachment security. *Child Development, 68,* 860–879.

Powell, B., Cooper, G., Hoffman, K., & Marvin, R. (2014). *The circle of security intervention: Enhancing attachment in early parent-child relationships*. New York: Guilford.

Riem, M., Bakermans-Kranenburg, M., van Ijzendoorn, M., Out, D., & Rombouts, S. (2012). Attachment in the brain: adult attachment representations predict amygdala and behavioral responses to infant crying. *Attachment & Human Development, 14*(6), 533–551.

Robertson, J. (Writer). (1953a). Film: A two-year-old goes to hospital: Concord Video and Film Council.

Robertson, J. (1953b). Some responses of young children to loss of maternal care. *Nursing Times, April*, 382–386.

Robertson, J. (Writer). (1971). Film: Thomas, aged two years four months, in foster care for ten days: Concord Video and Film Council.

Robertson, J., & Robertson, J. (1989). *Separation and the very young*. London: Free Association Books.

Sanders, M. (Producer). (2010). Professor Sanders discusses how Triple P helps promote secure attachment in children. http://www.psy.uq.edu.au/activity/media.html?mid=12. Accessed 7 July 2014.

Speltz, M., Greenberg, M., & DeKlyen, M. (1990). Attachment in preschoolers with disruptive behavior: A comparison of clinic-referred and nonproblem children. *Development and Psychopathology, 2,* 31–46.

Speltz, M., DeKlyen, M., Greenberg, M., & Dryden, M. (1995). Clinic referral for oppositional defiant disorder: Relative significance of attachment and behavioral variables. *Journal of Abnormal Child Psychology, 23*(4), 487–507.

Speltz, M., DeKlyen, M., & Greenberg, M. (1999). Attachment in boys with early onset conduct problems. *Development and Psychopathology, 11,* 269–285.

Steele, H., & Steele, M. (2008). *Clinical applications of the adult attachment interview*. New York: Guilford.

Stovall-McClough, K., & Cloitre, M. (2003). Reorganization of unresolved childhood traumatic memories following exposure therapy. *Annals of the New York Academy of Sciences, 2008,* 297–299.

Toth, S., Rogosch, F., Manly, J., & Cicchetti, D. (2006). The efficacy of toddler-parent psychotherapy to reorganize attachment in the young offspring of mothers with major depressive disorder: A randomized preventive trial. *Journal of Consulting and Clinical Psychology, 74,* 1006–1016.

Troutman, B., Arndt, S., Caspers, K., & Yucuis, R. (2010). *Infant negative emotionality moderates the association between quantity of nonfamilial day care and infant-mother attachment.* Paper presented at the Scientific Proceedings of the American Academy of Child & Adolescent Psychiatry's 57th Annual Meeting, New York, NY.

van den Boom, D. (1988). *Neonatal irritability and the development of attachment: Observation and intervention.* Dissertation, University of Leiden.

van den Boom, D. (1989). Neonatal irritability and the development of attachment. In G. Kohnstamm, J. Bates, & M. Rothbart (Eds.), *Temperament in childhood.* New York: Wiley.

van den Boom, D. (1994). The influence of temperament and mothering on attachment and exploration: An experimental manipulation of sensitive responsiveness among lower-class mothers with irritable infants. *Child Development, 65,* 1457–1477.

Van Ijzendoorn, M. (1995). Adult attachment representations, parental responsiveness, and infant attachment: A meta-analysis on the predictive validity of the adult attachment interview. *Psychological Bulletin, 117*(3), 387–403.

van IJzendoorn, M., & Hubbard, F. (2000). Are infant crying and maternal responsiveness during the first year related to infant-mother attachment at 15 months? *Attachment & Human Development, 2*(3), 371–391.

van Ijzendoorn, M., Schuengel, C., & Bakermans-Kranenberg, M. (1999). Disorganized attachment in early childhood: Meta-analysis of precursors, concomitants, and sequelae. *Development and Psychopathology, 11,* 225–249.

Zeanah, C., Berlin, L., & Boris, N. (2011). Practitioner review: Clinical applications of attachment theory and research for infants and young children. *The Journal of Child Psychology and Psychiatry, 52*(8), 819–833.

Beth Troutman PhD is a Clinical Professor in Psychiatry at the University of Iowa Carver College of Medicine. Her teaching, research, and clinical work has focused on improving parent-child interactions for more than 30 years. She has had a foot in more than one theoretical camp since graduate school, conducting research on parenting self-efficacy, temperament, and attachment theory and disseminating Parent-Child Interaction Therapy (PCIT), a behavioral model for improving parenting.

Chapter 3
Comparison of Attachment and Behavioral Parenting Perspectives

> *"Further study is needed to delineate how attachment and behavioral variables might best complement each other in illuminating the origins and development of disruptive behavior problems." (Speltz et al. 1995)*

Three-year-old Brodie's[1] *terrible twos had progressed to the even more terrible threes. He seemed to create chaos wherever he went. His favorite word was no, the dog ran away whenever he came near, he rarely slept through the night, threw epic tantrums, and was angry much of the time. Even something as simple as getting dressed in the morning became a pitched battle of wills between him and his mother, Maggie. Maggie, who had taken a leave from her successful career to stay at home with Brodie was counting the days until he started kindergarten. Maggie dreaded getting up in the morning to face another day of conflict with Brodie and thought back longingly on her days in the courtroom. She felt guilty about feeling this way and wondered whether her negative feelings about Brodie contributed to his problems. When her husband, Kendrick, returned home after a long day of work, Maggie was exhausted and he wondered what had happened to the beautiful, vivacious woman who had longed to be a mother. One night after Brodie had finally fallen asleep, they finally admitted to each other what they had only begun to admit to themselves—they were in over their heads. After surviving difficult childhoods to become successful professionals, they were failing at parenting. They vowed to put their considerable talents towards the goal of improving their parenting by finding out the best way to address Brodie's behavior problems. They made a list of people they knew with expertise on parenting, divided the list, and agreed to spend the next week gathering information about how to address Brodie's behavior problems.*

The following week, as they reviewed the information at their late night summit, they were amazed at the variability in the advice about the best way to manage Brodie's behavior problems. Maggie started with the advice from Paula, a stay-

[1] This is a fictional account written to illustrate popular parenting advice based on attachment and behavioral views of positive parenting.

B. Troutman, *Integrating Behaviorism and Attachment Theory in Parent Coaching*, SpringerBriefs in Psychology, DOI 10.1007/978-3-319-15239-4_3

at-home mother of a 1-year-old who practiced “attachment parenting”. Paula suggested Brodie’s behavior problems were the result of being weaned too early and noted Maggie seemed angry at Brodie. She recommended co-sleeping to improve their attachment relationship and warned against the use of time-outs. Maggie and Kendrick agreed you didn’t need to be a particularly astute observer to see that Maggie was angry at Brodie and having Brodie sleep with them was unlikely to decrease their anger towards him.

Next, they discussed the advice from Brian who noted behavioral interventions had the strongest empirical support for addressing children’s behavior problems. He recommended a book that emphasized the use of natural consequences to address children’s behavior problems and recommended time-outs for Brodie’s tantrums and misbehavior. This approach seemed promising and they liked that it had been researched but Maggie had experienced harsh, punitive parenting and was concerned Brodie might spend the entire day in time-out given the frequency of his tantrums and misbehavior.

Finally, they discussed Maggie’s conversation with Beatrice, a mother of four children ranging in age from adolescence through young adulthood. After hearing Maggie’s description of life with Brodie, Beatrice told Maggie her 16-year-old son had similar problems when he was Brodie’s age. She and her husband argued about the best approach and, in desperation, scheduled an evaluation with a therapist—not sure whether they or their son needed therapy. The therapist conducted an evaluation that included discussions of how they were parented and observations of their interactions with their son. Following the evaluation, Beatrice and her husband participated in play sessions with their child while the therapist coached them. Beatrice indicated the parent coaching focused on learning different ways of interpreting and responding to her son’s behavior. Beatrice said she knew it sounded like overkill to see a “baby shrink” to learn how to play with your child but the parent coaching had made a big difference in their family.

As Maggie and Kendrick discussed Beatrice’s story, they agreed the person who had failed to give them specific parenting advice had been the most helpful. Although they hadn’t yet identified the specific approach they would use, they had an idea for how to become better parents.

Comparison of Attachment and Behavioral Views of Parent-Child Interactions

The two theoretical models of parenting described in Chaps. 1 and 2 are often presented as a forced choice, with parents and providers needing to choose either an attachment-focused or behavioral-focused intervention. This seems to be especially true of parenting books and blogs aimed at parents where the differences between the two perspectives tend to be magnified, e.g. ‘Time-Outs’ Are Hurting Your Child” (Siegel and Bryson 2014).

Overlap between Attachment and Behavioral Assessments of Child-Parent Interactions

The few studies comparing attachment and behavioral assessments of parent-child interactions find relatively little overlap between the two types of assessments. Speltz et al. (1995) examined the association of attachment security, assessed using the modified Strange Situation Procedure (SSP) for preschoolers (Cassidy and Marvin, 1992; Main and Cassidy 1985), and frequency of maternal and child behaviors during child-led play, parent-led play, and toy clean-up assessed by the Dyadic Parent-Child Interaction Coding System (DPICS) (Eyberg and Robinson 1981; Robinson and Eyberg 1981). Out of 21 maternal behaviors examined (child-directed talk, critical statements, praise, commands, responds to deviant behavior, talking in role play, and positive/neutral physical contact) only one was statistically significant at the .01 level; maternal critical comments during toy clean-up (Speltz et al. 1995). Out of 15 child behaviors examined (descriptive comments, talking in role play, positive/neutral physical contact, deviant behavior, and compliance) only one was statistically significant at the .01 level; child deviant behavior during toy clean-up (Speltz et al. 1995). Notably, the parent and child behaviors correlated with attachment security occur during toy clean-up, a situation that places stress on the relationship. In two longitudinal studies, secure infant-parent attachment fails to predict power-assertive control (e.g. holding the child's hand firmly or taking away a toy) at 33 or 52 months (Kochanska and Kim 2012).

Predictive Validity of Attachment and Behavioral Assessments of Parent-Child Interactions

Surprisingly, given the preponderance of research on behavioral parenting interventions for disruptive behavior, the only study to compare the predictive validity of attachment and behavioral assessments found insecure child-mother attachment is a better predictor of whether a child is referred for disruptive behavior than frequency of maternal commands, maternal criticism, child deviant behavior and child noncompliance *combined* (Speltz et al. 1995). Child conduct problems are best predicted by a combination of power-assertive control and attachment security (Kochanska and Kim 2012).

Differences between Behavioral and Attachment Views of Positive Parenting

In the scientific literature, one reason for the differences between behavioral and attachment theory views of behavior is the influence of ethology on attachment theory. Bowlby was strongly influenced by ethology's view that patterns of behavior have evolved in conjunction with specific physical characteristics. For example, human infants are much less capable and more dependent on their caregivers than infants of other species. This contributes to both an extended period of dependency and a tendency to flee to a person rather than a place when faced with threats in the environment. Viewed from this perspective, one of the primary goals of the child-parent attachment relationship is protecting the child from dangerous situations and predators, including other humans.

Consequently, one of the areas of starkest contrast between behavioral and attachment parenting models of positive parenting involves response to distress. As noted in Chap. 2, attachment theory-based research indicates maternal responsiveness to distress is a significant predictor of secure attachment. Thus, from an attachment perspective, teaching parents to use ignoring and time-out from positive reinforcement to manage their child's behavior may undermine security of attachment by encouraging parents to ignore their child's distress.

Due to the difference in focus between behavioral and attachment views of optimal parent-child interactions, critics of attachment theory sometimes have the impression attachment theorists do not believe in parents setting limits on their child's behavior. This is not the case. Ainsworth (1967) notes the importance of young children learning about the limits of their power and not being able to control their parents. However, she also notes this lesson is best learned after the child has had the experience of being able to control his world by his parents responding to his signals and requests.

Differences Between Evidence-Based Attachment and Behavioral Interventions

As shown in Table 3.1, behavioral and attachment-based models differ in the child behaviors that are a focus of the intervention and the view of the positive parenting response to child behaviors. Attachment-based interventions primarily focus on improving sensitive responsiveness to distress signals such as fussing and crying while interventions based on behaviorism primarily focus on ignoring disruptive behavior such as yelling, sassing, and whining. Since only one of the interventions listed in Table 3.1 (van den Boom (1994)) uses detailed behavioral coding of the child behaviors that are a focus of the intervention, it is not possible to determine the degree of overlap between child behaviors viewed as attachment signals in attachment-based interventions and those viewed as disruptive behavior or tantrums in behavioral interventions.

Behavioral and attachment-based interventions shown in Table 3.1 focus on importance of physical contact but differ on when parents should use positive physical contact. Attachment-based interventions focus on parents using positive physical contact when their child is distressed while behavioral interventions focus on parents using positive physical contact when their child is exhibiting appropriate behavior.

Table 3.1 Examples of positive parent response to child behaviors in attachment and behavioral parenting interventions

Description of positive parent response to child behaviors	Population	Primary theoretical model/ Intervention	Reference
"Instances of fussing or crying served as targets for behavior change in sensitive responsiveness to negative infant signals." "If soothing did not occur, mothers were asked to soothe their infants, and the importance of soothing a crying infant was highlighted."	6-month-old infants in low income households selected for neonatal irritability and their biological mothers	Attachment (Skill-based parent coaching for mothers of irritable babies)	van den Boom 1994
"Attention-seeking behaviors (e.g. whining, nagging, temper tantrums, interrupting) can be ignored." "Decide ahead of time which "not OK" behaviors to ignore."	3- to 8-year-old children presenting with noncompliance	Behavioral (Helping the Noncompliant Child)	McMahon and Forehand 2003
"Some mothers worked on recognizing and responding sensitively to infant cues of distress more quickly, and others focused on allowing the infant to explore."	6-month-old infants in low income households and their biological mothers	Attachment (Circle of Security Home Visiting)	Cassidy et al. 2011
"Specifically, the therapist would help the parent ignore the infant when yelling and praise the infant for being calm and quiet as soon as the infant stopped yelling." "parents were especially encouraged to use positive physical touch (e.g. patting the infant's back) and nonverbal praise (e.g. clapping hands) along with verbal praise to enhance reinforcement for appropriate behaviors."	12- to 15-month-old infants in low income households and their biological mothers	Behavioral (Parent-Child Interaction Therapy (PCIT))	Bagner et al .2013
"Ignore his request for candy and his knocking over of the truck. Instead, get the other truck and begin to enthusiastically roll it on the floor, making an engine sound as you roll it."	23-month-old maltreated toddler and his biological mother	Behavioral (Parent-Child Attunement Therapy (PCAT))	Dombrowski et al. 2005

Table 3.1 (continued)

"Most importantly, parents were encouraged and supported in responding to their children's distress in the moment throughout the remaining sessions."	Parents of children between the ages of 1 and 21 months enrolled in a program to divert children from foster care due to identified needs such as domestic violence, parental substance abuse, and child neglect	Attachment (Attachment and Biobehavioral Catch-Up (ABC))	Bernard et al. 2012
"Ignoring can reduce children's *attention-seeking* behavior (yelling, sassing, whining, crying for no real reason)"	Children between the ages of 2 and 6 years, 11 months with disruptive behavior disorders, at risk for disruptive behavior disorders, or at risk for child abuse, and their caregivers	Behavioral (PCIT)	Eyberg and Funderburk 2011
"sensitivity involves: (a) responding to child distress signals with comfort and appropriate structuring and (b) promoting and supporting active child exploration when the child is not distressed."	Children between 12 and 71 months of age being monitored for child maltreatment and their primary caregiver (biological mother or father)	Attachment (Relationship Intervention Program)	Moss et al. 2011

Another component of behavioral interventions sometimes viewed as inconsistent with attachment theory is the use of time-out from positive reinforcement (Powell et al. 2014; Siegel and Bryson 2014). As with ignoring, this is based on differences in conceptualizations of positive parenting behavior. In terms of the negative impact of using time-out to discipline children, published research has failed to examine whether parents' use of time-out is associated with insecure attachment. National surveys conducted in the United States indicate 42–70% of parents of young children use time outs (Barkin et al. 2007; Regalado et al. 2004). Given the rate of secure attachment, this suggests at least some parents in securely attached dyads use time-outs with their child.

Similarities between Behavioral and Attachment-Based Parenting Interventions

When moving from theory to practice, it is clear there are a number of similarities between behavioral and attachment-based parenting interventions. As in most of the literature on psychosocial interventions, relatively few studies of parent-child interventions examine the mechanism leading to improvements. Thus, improvements may be due to similarities between behavioral and attachment-based parenting interventions.

One commonality between a number of behavioral and attachment-based parenting interventions is the focus on increasing play between children and parents. Thus, increasing the amount of time parents play with their child may be a core component of effective interventions for young children regardless of the theoretical approach guiding the intervention. A recent study of low income mothers compared behavioral coaching of child-led play (i.e. coaching mothers to praise and describe their child's play) to a "play-as-usual" control group where mothers were simply encouraged to play with their child as they usually would (Kochanska et al. 2013). In both groups, there were significant increases in children's cooperation with their mothers and the effect size for the play-as-usual group ($d=0.58$) was actually somewhat larger than the effect size for the child-led play group ($d=0.31$). Mother's ratings of their child's social-emotional competence also improved significantly in both groups (Kochanska et al. 2013).

Another similarity between behavioral- and attachment-oriented parenting interventions is a focus on improving parents' observational skills and reinforcing parents' positive parenting skills. Although a variety of different strategies and theoretical models are used to improve the parent's skills at observing their own behavior and their child's behavior, the core component may be improving the parent's observational skills by giving the parent a framework for observations and a supportive environment for making sense of these observations. In the Incredible Years and Triple P behavioral interventions, standard videos of parents handling different situations are used to facilitate observations of antecedents and responses to child behavior from a behavioral perspective. In Parent-Child Interaction Therapy (PCIT) and Helping the Noncompliant Child, parent's observational skills improve through describing their child's nonverbal behavior, reflecting their child's verbal behavior, and praising their child's nonverbal and verbal behavior. Watch, Wait, and Wonder (WWW) and Child Parent Psychotherapy (CPP) also build observational skills by having parents describe and reflect on their child's behavior during sessions. Watch, Wait, and Wonder also builds observational skills by having parents keep a diary describing what happened during play with their child. A number of the interventions based on attachment theory described in Chap. 2 videotape parent-child interactions and watch the videotape with parents in order to facilitate observations.

Conclusions

While there are significant areas of disagreement between behavioral and attachment theory views of positive parenting, there are also areas of commonality. Closer examination of some of the areas of disagreement indicates some of the differences may involve responses to different types of child behavior.

The remainder of this book focuses on the framework I use for integrating behaviorism and attachment theory in my work with families. Chapter 4 lays out a framework for coaching parents in behavior management skills and behaviors that promote attachment security. Chapters 5, 6, 7, and 8 are organized around tailoring coaching to different working models of attachment.

References

Ainsworth, M. (1967). *Infancy in Uganda*. Baltimore: Johns Hopkins Press.

Bagner, D., Rodriguez, G., Blake, C., & Rosa-Olivares, J. (2013). Home-based preventive parenting intervention for at-risk infants and their families: An open trial. *Cognitive and Behavioral Practice, 20,* 334–348.

Barkin, S., Scheindlin, B., Ip, E., Richardson, I., & Finch, S. (2007). Determinants of parental discipline practices: A national sample from primary care practices. *Clinical Pediatrics, 46*(1), 64–69.

Bernard, K., Dozier, M., Bick, J., Lewis-Morrarty, E., Lindhiem, O., & Carlson, E. (2012). Enhancing attachment organization among maltreated children: Results of a randomized clinical trial. *Child Development, 83*(2), 623–636.

Cassidy, J., & Marvin, R. (1992). *Attachment organization in three and four year olds: Coding manual*. Unpublished scoring manual.

Cassidy, J., Woodhouse, S., Sherman, L., Stupica, B., & Lejuez, C. W. (2011). Enhancing infant attachment security: An examination of treatment efficacy and differential susceptibility. *Development and Psychopathology, 23,* 131–148.

Dombrowski, S., Timmer, S., Blacker, D., & Urquiza, A. (2005). A positive behavioural intervention for toddlers: Parent-child attunement therapy. *Child Abuse Review, 14,* 132–151.

Eyberg, S., & Funderburk, B. (2011). *Parent-child interaction therapy protocol*. Gainesville: PCIT International, Inc.

Eyberg, S., & Robinson, E. (1981). *Dyadic parent-child interaction coding system*. Unpublished coding manual.

Kochanska, G., & Kim, S. (2012). Toward a new understanding of legacy of early attachments for future antisocial trajectories: Evidence from two longitudinal studies. *Development and Psychopathology, 24,* 783–806.

Kochanska, G., Kim, S., Boldt, L., & Nordling, J. (2013). Promoting toddlers' positive social-emotional outcomes in low-income families: A play-based experimental study. *Journal of Clinical Child & Adolescent Psychology, 42*(5), 700–712.

Main, M., & Cassidy, J. (1985). Assessments of child-parent attachment at six years of age. Unpublished manuscript.

McMahon, R., & Forehand, R. (2003). *Helping the noncompliant child: Family-based treatment for oppositional behavior* (2nd ed.). New York: Guilford.

Moss, E., Dubois-Comtois, K., Cyr, C., St-Laurent, D., & Bernier, A. (2011). Efficacy of a home-visiting intervention aimed at improving maternal sensitivity, child attachment, and behavioral outcomes for maltreated children: A randomized control trial. *Development and Psychopathology, 23,* 195–210.

Powell, B., Cooper, G., Hoffman, K., & Marvin, R. (2014). *The circle of security intervention: Enhancing attachment in early parent-child relationships*. New York: Guilford.

Regalado, M., Sareen, H., Inkelas, M., Wissow, L., & Halfon, N. (2004). Parents' discipline of young children: Results from the national survery of early childhood health. *Pediatrics, 113*(6), 1952–1958.

Robinson, E., & Eyberg, S. (1981). The dyadic parent-child interaction coding system: Standardization and validation. *Journal of Consulting and Clinical Psychology, 49*(2), 245–250.

Siegel, D., & Bryson, T. (2014). 'Time-Outs' are hurting your child. http://time.com/3404701/discipline-time-out-is-not-good/#3404701/discipline-time-out-is-not-good/. Accessed 18 Oct 2014.

Speltz, M., DeKlyen, M., Greenberg, M., & Dryden, M. (1995). Clinic referral for oppositional defiant disorder: Relative significance of attachment and behavioral variables. *Journal of Abnormal Child Psychology, 23*(4), 487–507.

van den Boom, D. (1994). The influence of temperament and mothering on attachment and exploration: An experimental manipulation of sensitive responsiveness among lower-class mothers with irritable infants. *Child Development, 65,* 1457–1477.

Beth Troutman PhD is a Clinical Professor in Psychiatry at the University of Iowa Carver College of Medicine. Her teaching, research, and clinical work has focused on improving parent-child interactions for more than 30 years. She has had a foot in more than one theoretical camp since graduate school, conducting research on parenting self-efficacy, temperament, and attachment theory and disseminating Parent-Child Interaction Therapy (PCIT), a behavioral model for improving parenting.

Part II
Integrated Model for Coaching Positive Parenting

Chapter 4
Framework for Integrating Behaviorism and Attachment Theory in Parent Coaching

Synergy: The interaction or cooperation of two or more organizations, substances, or other agents to produce a combined effect greater than the sum of their separate effects. (Oxford English Dictionary 2014)

When the therapist heard the brusque voice mail from a mother indicating she was potentially interested in her services but wanted to know more about the therapist's credentials before scheduling an appointment, she dreaded returning the call. The therapist already felt evaluated and potentially criticized by the tone in the voice mail. She realized the voice mail reminded her of her 4th grade teacher who always seemed to know when she had forgotten to do her homework. When the therapist returned the call to Maggie, her reaction softened as she heard the desperation in Maggie's voice describing her son Brodie's tantrums, noncompliance, and anger[1]*. The therapist described her credentials and experience to Maggie and explained her approach to working with families. She described the intake session where she would talk with Maggie and her husband, Kendrick, and the initial parent-child evaluation session where she would observe Maggie and Kendrick interacting with Brodie.*

At the initial intake, Maggie and Kendrick described Brodie's behavior problems and the strategies they had tried to address them. When asked about how they had been disciplined as children, they spoke openly and poignantly about their childhoods. They had both grown up poor and wanted to offer better opportunities to their children. They worked hard and succeeded in their careers, waiting until they were financially stable to have a child. Maggie became tearful as she described her parents' high expectations and liberal use of spanking to enforce those expectations. Although she had resolved not to spank her own children, she had begun to wonder whether Brodie's behavior problems were the result of being too lenient and "waiting too long to have children". Kendrick described his parents as "disciplining

[1] This is a fictional account written to illustrate an evaluation of parent-child interactions utilizing assessments based on attachment theory and behaviorism.

B. Troutman, *Integrating Behaviorism and Attachment Theory in Parent Coaching*, SpringerBriefs in Psychology, DOI 10.1007/978-3-319-15239-4_4

through guilt". He described an incident he remembered where his parents talked with him about hitting his little sister. They explained that hitting was not acceptable in their family, talked about how important he was to his little sister and how it made her feel to be hit by her big brother, and told him how disappointed they were in him.

At the end of the intake, the therapist reassured Maggie and Kendrick she had worked with other families with similar problems. She told them she was confident they would be able to improve their relationship with Brodie and address his behavior problems. The therapist then described the standardized observations that would be the focus of the next session—the observation of parent-child interactions. Maggie and Kendrick expressed concern that Brodie would be a perfect angel during the evaluation. The therapist told Maggie and Kendrick she was not likely to see the types of behavior problems seen in their home but, nevertheless, the standardized situations would provide useful information that would be helpful in planning how to address his behavior problems.

When the therapist entered the waiting room for the parent-child evaluation, Brodie was living up to his reputation, pounding on the table with his fist while looking at his parents for a reaction. After introducing herself to Brodie, the therapist told him they would be going to the play room where there were more toys. Brodie jumped up and eagerly tugged on his father's hand. After entering the play room, the therapist explained to Brodie that she would be talking to his parents through a bug-in-the-ear while they played with him. Brodie headed to the parking ramp toy on the floor while his mother put in the listening device and his father returned to the waiting room to wait his turn. Brodie began pushing cars down the ramp while his mother went and sat in a nearby chair. After playing for 5 min, the therapist told his mother through the bug-in-the-ear to leave the room. Brodie initially argued with his mother about her need to leave the room but when she firmly told him he needed to stay, he returned to playing and stayed in the room for the 5 min separation. Brodie continued to push cars down the ramp, humming softly to himself and occasionally looking at the door. When his mother returned, he said "Look. I go down the ramp fast". "Just like your father" Maggie said smiling. Interactions between Brodie and his mother continued to go smoothly through a second 5 min separation, 5 min reunion, and 5 min of child-led play.

When told to engage Brodie in parent-led play, the therapist recognized the brusque tone of voice she had heard in Maggie's voice mail and the demanding, obnoxious child she had met in the waiting room. Maggie and Brodie's interactions became increasingly negative and the therapist noted a knot in her stomach as they headed into the clean-up situation. When told to have Brodie clean up the toys, Maggie's tone changed from brusque to drill sergeant. The therapist would not have been the least bit surprised if Maggie had told Brodie to drop and give her 10. Brodie eventually slammed a block in the container and Maggie barked "Softly!". At the end of 5 min, the therapist took a deep breath and walked in the room.

After a brief break, Kendrick and Brodie entered the play room. Brodie yelled "Tractors!" and ran over to explore the tractors the therapist had placed on the table. Kendrick beamed at Brodie's enthusiasm and told the therapist "Brodie loves tractors." Kendrick and Brodie played and chatted about tractors for the next 5 min. When it came time for the separation, Kendrick told Brodie he needed to step out for a couple of minutes and Brodie needed to "stay and take care of the farm." Brodie continued to hook and unhook equipment to the tractor. When Kendrick returned, Brodie smiled and began telling his father what he had done. Kendrick was delighted at Brodie's correct labeling of the combine and baler. The second separation and reunion were similar to the first with Brodie playing quietly when by himself and returning to joint play when his father returned. The good will continued through the child-led play and the therapist noticed she was smiling at the heartwarming interactions between Brodie and his father. The therapist noticed herself feeling tense and hating to interrupt the positive interactions when she signaled Kendrick to begin parent-directed interaction. Kendrick said "Hey Bud. We've played with tractors a long time. How about we build something with the blocks?". Much to the therapist's surprise, Brodie readily agreed and began building blocks with his father. When the therapist told the father to have Brodie pick up the toys 5 min later, she was even more surprised when Brodie immediately complied with picking up the toys as he and his father sang the clean up song.

Assessment of Parent-Child Interactions

Prior to beginning treatment, I conduct an assessment that routinely includes an intake interview, standardized assessments of parent-child interactions, and standardized assessments of the child's behavior problems. (I include additional standardized assessments as needed to address presenting concerns, e.g. school behavior checklists and cognitive testing if the child is having problems at school.) I view parent-child interactions through both an attachment and behavioral lens beginning with the initial assessment. Since there is relatively little overlap between attachment and behavioral assessments, I find this is easiest to do by including both types of assessments. The research-based assessments of parent-child interactions I conduct are based on attachment theory [Strange Situation Procedure or modified Strange Situation Procedure for Preschoolers (Cassidy et al. 1992)] and behaviorism [(Dyadic Parent-Child Interaction Coding System) (Eyberg et al. 2005, 2013)]. I also have the parents complete questionnaires about the child's behavior problems and social-emotional functioning [Child Behavior Checklist (CBCL) (Achenbach 2000) and Eyberg Child Behavior Inventory (ECBI) (Eyberg and Pincus 1999)]. When the presenting concern involves attachment or attachment disorder, I include additional research-based assessments of attachment such as the Disturbances of Attachment Interview, (Smyke, Dumitrescu, and Zeanah, 2002) Circle of Security Interview (Main and Goldwyn, 1998; Hoffman et al. 2006; Powell et al. 2014), and/or Adult Attachment Interview (Steele and Steele 2008). This pre-treatment assessment is used to tailor parent coaching to presenting concerns and working models of attachment.

In the hypothetical case of Brodie, Kendrick, and Maggie, the ECBI completed by Kendrick and Maggie indicates Brodie is exhibiting significant disruptive behavior with parents' T scores on the intensity and problem scales both above 70 (i.e. more than 2 SD above the mean). CBCLs completed by both parents indicate in addition to significant externalizing behavior problems (T scores > 70), Brodie is more anxious and unhappy than other boys his age (internalizing problems T scores > 60). The behavioral observations of Brodie and his parents provide information about the family's significant strengths as well as the areas where they struggle. First, observations of Brodie's reactions to separations and reunions with his parents indicate their relationship allows him to use his parents as a secure base as well as a haven of safety, i.e. the overall quality of their attachment relationship is secure. However, the observations of Brodie in the waiting room and during parent-led play and clean-up with his mother also indicate significant problems with compliance and the use of misbehavior to escape from demands.

Countertransference

I define countertransference as the ways in which providers respond to the families they advise. I use this term to refer to both the feelings interventionists have towards parents and children and the ways they behave towards them. Rather than viewing countertransference as something that needs to be "managed", I view it as providing useful information. In order for countertransference to provide useful information about the family, it is important I be able to reflect on my emotional and behavioral reactions and factors influencing my reactions. In other words, my reactions are most useful when I am able to sort out what aspects of my reactions reflect the parent and child's internal working models of attachment and reinforcement history and what aspects reflect my internal working model of attachment and reinforcement history. When I am able to view my reactions through this lens, it provides both general information (i.e. how other people are likely to respond to this parent and child) and specific information (i.e. the types of negative interaction patterns I may fall into with the family). This makes it easier to engage the family and avoid replicating previous negative interactional patterns.

In the hypothetical case of Brodie, Maggie, and Kendrick, the therapist's reflections on her reactions to the family provide some clues about the family's struggles. The therapist reflected on several instances where she felt tense and defensive during interactions with Maggie. When she reflected on these moments, she realized they typically occurred when Maggie was being brusque and these were moments where Maggie likely felt vulnerable or inadequate. Given Maggie's concern about being too lenient, the therapist guessed Maggie did not recognize how confrontational she appeared to Brodie or others in these moments. The therapist reflected on how differently she felt when observing the warm, relaxed interactions between Brodie and Kendrick and Brodie's compliance with his father's indirect commands.

The therapist recognized this as a positive sign since it indicated Brodie had not internalized a sense of himself as "naughty". However, when she looked at it from Maggie's perspective, she suspected it contributed to Maggie's sense of inadequacy. She also suspected Maggie's tendency to cover up her feelings of vulnerability with brusqueness was due to her difficulty sharing feelings of vulnerability.

Why Parent Coaching?

A number of the interventions described in Chaps. 1 and 2 involve coaching parents—either in vivo as they interact with their child, through video review of their interactions with their child, or through a combination of the two coaching approaches. Parenting seems to be one of those skills where a coaching approach is especially applicable. Parenting involves procedural memory, i.e. learning how to do something. In that way, it is similar to learning to drive a car or play a sport. Thus, the opportunity to be coached in parenting, either in vivo while interacting with one's child or through discussing and analyzing videos of responses to one's child, seems an especially fruitful way to learn a different way of responding. In addition, parenting evokes strong emotions. In the face of these strong emotions, parents may revert to previously learned ways of responding despite "knowing better". For those of us who learned to drive prior to anti-lock braking systems, it is similar to the automatic tendency to pump the brakes in a stressful situation such as bad weather/slick roads even though we "know" we have anti-lock brakes and should not pump. During parent coaching we are able to help a parent recognize and override these automatic tendencies in emotional situations.

Incorporating Attachment Coaching into Behavioral Parent Coaching

Comments on the balance between attachment and exploration in healthy attachment, the child's attachment and exploration signals, and parenting behaviors associated with secure attachment can be incorporated into behavioral parent coaching when therapists recognize these behaviors. For example, comments can be incorporated into Hanf-based behavioral parent coaching approaches such as Helping the Noncompliant Child (Forehand and McMahon 1981; McMahon and Forehand 2003) or Parent-Child Interaction Therapy (PCIT) (Eyberg and Funderburk 2011; McNeil and Hembree-Kigin 2010; Urquiza et al. 2011) where parents are being coached to use behavioral parenting skills to facilitate positive parent-child interaction during child-led play (Child's Game or Child-Directed Interaction) and parent-led play (Parent's Game or Parent-Directed Interaction).

Attachment-informed Approach to Coaching Ignoring during Behavioral Child-Led Play

As noted in Chap. 3, from an attachment perspective the potential risk of ignoring is the parent will ignore attachment signals and undermine the security of the attachment relationship. I coach ignoring judiciously. My coaching focuses on parents using ignoring in the context of child-led play with their child. I rarely recommend parents use ignoring outside of this context. Consistent with the Helping the Noncompliant Child approach to child-led play (McMahon and Forehand 2003), I work to develop a shared definition with the parent of specific behaviors to ignore prior to coaching the parent. When helping parents define which behaviors to ignore, I am guided by the parent's concerns and the child's current level of behavior problems. However, I also use my training in attachment theory to guide parents away from ignoring certain behaviors. For example, I am uncomfortable with parents trying to determine whether crying is "attention-seeking" or "for no good reason" so I do not coach parents to ignore crying. When coaching ignoring, I tend to focus on behaviors such as playing roughly with toys or whining that are not likely to be confused with attachment signals or be indicative of distress.

One of the "behaviors" parents often talk about trying to ignore is tantrums (also referred to as emotional outbursts, hissy fits, and meltdowns). Although it is often assumed providers and parents are talking about the same behavior when they use these terms, I find there are vastly different definitions of tantrum or meltdown. Thus, if tantrums are one of the behaviors parents want to address, it is especially important to carefully explore their definition of tantrums. When trying to help parents better define tantrums, I sometimes find it useful to share the distinction between "distress tantrums" where the child needs help handling strong emotions and "little Nero tantrums" where the child is using the tantrum behavior to bully the parent into behaving in a certain way (e.g. letting them have cookies at the store) (Sunderland 2006). Although young children often display emotional outbursts with features of both "distress" and "little Nero" tantrums, I find discussing this distinction with parents gives us a shorthand to begin discussing different aspects of tantrums as we move towards a shared definition. With some parents, I share Greg Prembroke's "Reasons My Kid Is Crying" book (Pembroke 2014) and web site: www.reasonsmysoniscrying.com when discussing tantrums as a way of discussing the different perspectives of young children and parents that can lead to conflict and distress.

If I do recommend parents use ignoring outside of child-led play, it is targeted to a particular, carefully defined behavior. From both an attachment and a behavioral perspective, ignoring is most effective when used rarely.

Although my primary focus is coaching parents to ignore misbehavior, I also coach some parents to ignore some expressions of frustration or minor distress. I conceptualize this type of ignoring in terms of how parents in securely attached dyads help their children learn self-regulation by supporting their emerging regulatory abilities. As noted in Chap. 2, sensitive responsiveness involves providing the "just right" amount of responsiveness to the child's distress (Beebe et al. 2010; van IJzendoorn and Hubbard 2000) as the child begins to develop skills in self-regulation.

The way I explain this to parents is "it is easier to learn to calm down when you are a little frustrated than it is when you are really angry. The more practice children have in calming down when they are a little upset, the less likely they will escalate to the point of being really upset." In PCIT, parents use a specific strategy when ignoring where they describe their own play. By describing their own play, the parent distracts the child and also communicates she is still present and available even if she is not interacting directly with the child. After parents become more comfortable with this strategy, they can also be coached to model strategies for coping with feelings such as describing how they are feeling or taking a deep breath while describing their own play.

I also use the concepts of shaping and differential reinforcement of other behavior when coaching parents in ignoring; the goal is for children to learn ways to engage their parents that are more adaptive than their current behaviors, not to engage in perfect behavior. For example, the first time I coach a parent whose child frequently yells at them, I coach the parent to describe her own play until he says something at a slightly lower decibel level. If he says "I'm mad", I would coach the parent to praise the child for using his words to tell her how he was feeling. Several parents have told me the most helpful part of being coached in ignoring was having someone tell them when to *stop* ignoring and focus on their child again.

Commenting on Attachment during Child-Led Play

Examples of in vivo coaching statements describing the child's signals for attachment or exploration are listed in Table 4.1. Just describing these signals is an important intervention. In the busy, sleep-deprived lives of parents raising young children, it is easy to miss the sweet moments that occur when interacting with a demanding preschooler. When coaching child-led play, we are able to slow down the world enough to help the parent notice and appreciate these moments. Even busy, sleep-deprived therapists can't help but be delighted when a young child hands the purple car to the parent saying "Purple is your favorite".

Parent coaches are also able to help parents see the impact of their behavior on their child by making observations about the positive impact of the parent's response. Examples of coaching statements that highlight parenting behaviors associated with secure attachment are shown in Table 4.2. The most challenging type of parent coaching is in vivo parent coaching where parents are coached to use new ways of responding to their child. These coaching statements need to be used sparingly and with the parent's working model of attachment in mind (see Chaps. 5–8). Examples of this type of coaching statement are listed in Table 4.3.

Table 4.1 Examples of in vivo coaching statements describing child's signals for attachment or exploration

That's his "mom smile". (attachment)
She let you have the princess doll. (attachment)
He really values your attention. (attachment)
She has decided to try something new today. (exploration)
He came over to play near you. (attachment)
I love the way he casually leans against you. (attachment)
He is enjoying building with those blocks. (exploration)
He needs his dad to check out that loose tooth. (attachment)
She lights up when she sees you. (attachment)
He loves that he did that on his own. (exploration)
He loves sharing his excitement with you. (attachment)
She moved closer to you. (attachment)
She is so proud of herself for building that on her own. (exploration)

Table 4.2 Examples of observations of parent behaviors that facilitate secure attachment

I love how you matched her excitement. (attunement)
You understand that he just needs to cuddle and have a little down time before playing today. (attunement)
Describing his play helps him be more independent. (providing secure base)
It's nice to see you enjoy a quiet moment together. (attunement)
You're on his wave length. (attunement)
That hug helps him calm down and go back to playing. (providing safe haven)

Table 4.3 Examples of coaching parent to respond differently during in vivo coaching

Child throws a toy. Parent says "Be careful. Stop treating the toys that way." Coach says to parent: "Go ahead and give him a command to put that toy in the box"
Child is building a zoo and puts the zebras and lions in the same pen. Parent moves zebras while saying to child: "You can't put the zebras and lions together. The lions will eat the zebras." Coach says to parent: "It's his zoo. Maybe in his zoo, lions don't eat zebras. Go ahead and describe what he's doing"

Video Feedback Parent Coaching Sessions

I use video feedback sessions with parents to help parents see the impact of their behavior on their child and address their perceptions of their child. These sessions are scheduled without the child present so the parent and I have a chance to discuss the interactions and their emotional responses without distraction. Watching yourself interacting with your child on video can be extremely stressful for parents. Parents may become defensive so it is important to move slowly and have a good working alliance with the parent. I set up the video review to be as relaxed and nonthreaten-

Table 4.4 Examples of coaching parent to examine their perceptions or respond differently during video feedback sessions

Do you remember this moment?
Do you notice anything now you didn't notice at the time?
What do you notice about your child?
What do you notice about your reaction?
Like post-game reviews, you can always see ways you might have responded differently when you watch tapes of interactions. Do you see anything where you wish you had responded differently?

ing as possible. I set up the room for video review sessions with a table with drinks and snacks between the parent and I with both of us facing the television screen. Initial video feedback sessions focus on pointing out the positive impact of their behavior on their child and moments of mutual enjoyment. I often make the same types of statements I make during in vivo coaching (see Tables 4.1 and 4.2). However, since I have the luxury of not having a busy, disruptive young child present, I am also able to find out about the parent's perception of the interactions.

I find it especially important to reflect on my countertransference reactions to the parent prior to these video sessions. My initial inclination in doing video review was to show parents the interactions I found problematic. I have learned that parents tend to be much harder on themselves than I am on them. It is important for me to provide a supportive environment and recognize their strengths as parents so they are able to feel safe enough to look at the areas where they struggle. I also find video feedback sessions helpful in remaining supportive and compassionate towards the parent. The parent's perceptions of the interactions gives me a small window into their view of relationships.

In later video feedback sessions, I begin to have parents look at how to improve their behavioral parenting skills—e.g. lost opportunities for praise or reflection. Once parents are more comfortable with the video feedback sessions, I begin asking questions designed to help parents identify their feelings during the interaction and how those feelings may have colored their perceptions and response to the child. Examples of the types of questions or prompts I might use in a video feedback session to encourage parents to examine their emotional responses are listed in Table 4.4. Video review often serves as a jumping off point for parents to discuss barriers to improving their interactions with their child such as feelings about how they were parented or their feelings about their child.

"Behavioral Countertransference" in Parent Coaching of Child-Led Play

Given their focus on behavior, countertransference is not a term typically used by behaviorists. However, from a behavioral perspective, parents are reinforcing, punishing, and shaping our interactions with them just as we are reinforcing, punishing, and shaping their behavior with us and their child. This section provides a framework for understanding and addressing this "behavioral countertransference".

When coaching parents in behavioral parenting skills, the goal is to use the same skills with parents they are being coached to use with their children (Eyberg 2005; Eyberg and Funderburk 2011; McNeil and Hembree-Kigin 2010). That is, when coaching parents in child-led play, behavioral parent coaches strive to primarily use positive reinforcement and differential attention—i.e. noticing and praising the parent's use of positive behavioral parenting skills.

Despite this emphasis, there seems to be a strong pull for behavioral parent coaches to become more directive and critical of parents over time, especially when the primary focus is getting parents to master specific skills. In an analogue study with a community sample, parents who receive "constructive criticism" (criticizing parents' use of negative parent behaviors and describing parents' use of positive parent behaviors) demonstrate significantly more positive parenting skills after 20 min of coaching than parents who receive only positive or neutral feedback (Herschell et al. 2008). Thus, in the short-term, therapists are reinforced for providing more critical feedback to parents by the parent's improvement in skill acquisition—just as parents are reinforced for criticizing their child by short-term improvement in their child's behavior.

Consistent with the idea that behavioral therapists are likely to be more directive than responsive during their coaching, a study of parent coaching of child-led play sessions in Parent-Child Interaction Therapy (PCIT) found therapists gave significantly more directive than responsive coaching statements (Barnett et al. 2014). This study also indicates how the therapist's coaching is impacted by the parent's behavior. Parents who praise their child more receive a greater number of responsive coaching comments (primarily praise) while parents with more deficits in child-led play skills receive more directive comments (Barnett et al. 2014). Thirteen percent of the parents in this study failed to return for a subsequent coaching session. For the families who did return for another coaching session, responsive coaching comments were associated with their use of labeled praises in the subsequent coaching session.

Research on attrition in PCIT indicates mothers who praise their child more and criticize them less at pre-treatment are more likely to complete PCIT (Fernandez and Eyberg 2009; Werba et al. 2006). It is easy to see why parents who praise their child more at the beginning of behavioral parent coaching are more likely to successfully complete treatment. The parent praises the child, the therapist praises the parent, and a cycle of responsive, positive reinforcement is quickly established. However, what about the families who at the beginning of treatment are praising their child less and criticizing them more? The relatively high drop-out rate in behavioral parenting interventions and research indicating parents are more resistant to implementing behavioral parenting skills when therapists are more directive (Patterson and Forgatch 1985) suggests behavioral therapists are becoming caught up in the "coercive cycle" (Patterson 1982) that characterizes many of the families referred for behavioral parenting interventions.

Table 4.5 Coding parent coaching during child-led play

	Tally	Number
Miscellaneous positive responsive coaching statement		
Describing child's behavior		
Describing or praising specific positive parenting behavior		
Educating parent about long-term impact of specific positive parenting behavior		
Observing impact of specific positive parenting behavior on child		
Making supportive/empathic statements acknowledging struggles		
Subtotal positive responsive statements		
Questions		
Indirect commands		
Direct commands		
Subtotal directive statements		
Criticism		
Total talk		
Subtotal Positive Responsive/Total Talk	(% Positive responsive)	
Subtotal Directive/Total Talk	(% Directive)	
Criticism/Total Talk	(% Criticism)	
Synchronous coaching	*Satisfactory*	*Needs practice*

In coaching parents, I find it helpful to remember the distinction made in the Adult Attachment Interview (AAI) between showing and telling. When coaching parents, it is important that what we are showing them during our coaching is the same as what we are telling them. For example, if we are telling parents to be positive and responsive to their children, we need to be positive and responsive to them. It is especially important to establish a high rate of responsive, positive coaching with parents who are not yet exhibiting a high rate of positive behavior towards their child. In fact, I think it is probably more important for these parents to experience responsive, positive coaching given their risk of dropping out of treatment (Fernandez and Eyberg 2009) and the likelihood they do not have much experience with positive, responsive relationships. I try to follow Pawl and St. John's (1998) "platinum rule" during coaching; "Do unto others as you would have others do unto others."

A form for coding parent coaching during child-led play is displayed in Table 4.5. Having a method for tracking my coaching helps me guard against "behavioral countertransference" drift by allowing me to evaluate whether what I am "showing" parents during coaching is the same as what I am "telling" them. My goal is for at least 80 % of my coaching statements to be positive and responsive. For some parents, I aim for an even higher rate of positive responsive coaching in order to counteract the parent's tendency to be directive and critical with their child. (Table 4.6)

Table 4.6 Definitions and examples of parent coaching during child-led play

Positive responsive coaching statements that do not fall into other categories
E.g. "Cool!" "He is so smart." "I love your new haircut."
Describing child's behavior
Describing behavior parent could attend to using positive behavioral parenting skill
E.g. "He is being very gentle with the blocks."
Describing balance between secure base and safe haven behavior
E.g. "She went out to explore and now she is back to check in."
Describing or praising specific positive parenting behavior
Describing or praising positive behavioral parenting skill
E.g. "Nice behavioral description."
Describing or praising parent's response to attachment signals
E.g. "I'm glad you helped him calm after he bumped himself."
Educating parent about long-term impact of positive parenting
Educating parent about effect a positive behavioral parenting skill could have on future behavior
E.g. "Describing what he is doing helps his attention span."
Educating parent about effect response to attachment or exploration signals could have on future behavior
E.g. "Letting him do that on his own will improve his self-confidence."
Educating parent about why you told them to do something
E.g. "I wanted you to describe your own play because he was playing rough with the toys."
Observing impact of specific positive parenting behavior on child
Observations of in session impact of positive behavioral parenting skill on child
E.g. "He just shared with you because you praised sharing earlier."
Observations of in session impact of parent's response to attachment signals
E.g. "After he leaned against you and you rubbed his head, he seemed ready to tackle that puzzle again."
Making supportive/empathic statements acknowledging struggles
Statements acknowledging parents' concerns
E.g. "I see what you mean about how he pushes limits." "You are usually so busy managing his behavior you don't get a chance to enjoy him."
Empathic statements acknowledging difficult moments during the session
E.g. "I know it must be hard to hear him say mean things to you."
Statements acknowledging parent's struggles with skills
E.g. "I know it is really hard not to ask questions." "It is really hard to describe his efforts and not jump in and solve it for him."
Questions
Prompt to use behavioral parenting skills
E.g. "What could you do instead of saying "stop"?"
Prompt to examine typical parenting response
E.g. "Would it be okay if he didn't match colors in his tower?"

Table 4.6 (continued)

Prompt to respond to attachment signal
E.g. "Do you think he wants to check in ?"
Indirect command
Indirect command suggesting parent use behavioral parenting skills or respond to attachment signals
E.g. "You can go ahead and pick him up. I didn't want you to think you needed to ignore his crying when he bumped his head."
Direct command
Direct command telling parent to use behavioral parenting skills or respond to attachment signals
E.g. "Pick up a toy and start describing your own play." "Sit back and let him lead the play."
Criticism
Criticizing parent's behavior or response to child
E.g. "Ouch. That sounded harsh." "It's important not to criticize your child."
Synchronous coaching
Therapist and parent appear to have a comfortable rhythm. There are neither long periods of uncomfortable silence nor too much talk

Attachment-Informed Approach to Coaching Compliance Training and Time-Out from Positive Reinforcement during Parent-Led Play

In the goal-directed partnership that characterizes healthy parent-child attachment, parents must set limits. In behavioral parent management approaches that evolved from the Hanf model, the second phase of treatment involves teaching the parent strategies for improving the child's compliance with parent demands and using time-out from positive reinforcement for noncompliance and aggression. Attachment relationships between parents and young children are hierarchical. Parents need to be in charge in order to protect children, one of the primary functions the child-parent attachment relationship evolved to provide. As stated succinctly by the developers of Circle of Security, parents need to be "bigger, stronger, wiser, and kind" (Powell et al. 2014).

Compliance training and time-out from positive reinforcement is a strategy for helping parents learn to be in charge in a calm, authoritative manner. Coaching parent-led interactions provides an opportunity to build the child's capacity to follow the parent's directions and the parent's capacity to be in charge. Compliance training and time-out from positive reinforcement can also be viewed as an extension of the focus on co-regulation begun during child-led play. Just as it is easier for a child to learn to manage frustration when he is a little frustrated, it is easier for a child to learn to follow directions when she is relatively calm, the parent's expectations are clear, and the parent's expectations are relatively easy to follow.

I often use the following metaphor to explain this phase to parents. "What if we taught children to read the same way we teach them to follow directions? What if we waited until both the child and the teacher were upset, handed them a chapter book, and told the teacher to make the child read it? This is often how parents and teachers try to discipline children who have difficulty following directions or become aggressive when upset. We wait until everyone is stressed and upset and then try to "teach them a lesson". Discipline means to teach and most of us have more difficulty learning and teaching when we are very upset. We are going to teach your child to follow directions and take time-outs when you are both relatively calm. This will make it easier for your child to learn these skills and for you to help him learn these skills. Once your child is better at following directions, it will be easier for you to help teach him other strategies when he becomes upset or aggressive. Just as we break it down into smaller steps to teach children to read, we are going to break down learning to follow directions into smaller steps. One of the first steps in learning to read is learning the A, B, Cs. We make it more fun for children to learn the alphabet by making it into a song. Similarly, we are going to have your child start learning to follow directions in a play situation where they have to follow little play commands while playing with you." When talking with parents about the use of time-out from positive reinforcement for managing children's noncompliance and aggression, I talk with them about what aspect of learning the parent-led play skills they expect to be most difficult and specifically ask them "What do you think will be the most difficult thing to hear your child say while in time-out?" Often these statements relate to their own experiences of being disciplined as a child or to their concerns about their child's perception of them.

As with ignoring, it is important to discuss with parents the specific child behaviors that will result in a time-out. Ainsworth's initial longitudinal study in Uganda (1967) suggests some parents in securely attached dyads make a distinction between distress and anger and respond differently to these emotional expressions. The majority of mothers in her Uganda sample responded the same way to their baby's angry tantrums as they did to their crying; i.e. mothers in securely attached dyads usually picked their babies up and comforted them when they cried and when they were angry. However, some mothers in securely attached dyads made a distinction between crying and anger—picking up their infants and soothing them when they were distressed, ignoring angry tantrums, and punishing them for anger expressed in aggressive behavior such as hitting. In evidence-based behavioral parent training models, time-outs are typically only given for noncompliance to a direct command following a warning and disobeying a house rule (typically aggression).

If parents ask about the use of ignoring or time-outs for "tantrums" or "meltdowns", I try to: (1) be clear about their behavioral definition of tantrums or meltdowns, (2) find out how often the child is having tantrums or meltdowns; (3) find out how long the tantrums or meltdowns last, and (4) identify antecedents of the tantrums or meltdowns (often it is transitions or being told no). Typically, we are able to identify strategies to address these behaviors that are likely to be more effective than ignoring or time-outs. One potential strategy is "time-ins" where parents

Table 4.7 Examples of in vivo coaching statements reinforcing positive impact on child of parent being calmly in charge

It will feel like a safer world to her when she trusts you are in charge
He followed directions because he wants to please you
She listens to you because she trusts you know what is best for her
It took everything he had to pick up the toys. He did it because he knew it was important to you
You understand how hard it is for her to follow directions but how being able to follow directions will help her do better in school

sit with the child and help him put words to their feelings (Powell et al. 2014; Siegel and Bryson 2014). Time-ins are sometimes recommended as an alternative to time-outs (Siegel and Bryson 2014) and may be useful when a child is upset and the parent is able to remain calm and help the child identify their feelings. However, I do not recommend using time-ins for noncompliance or aggression.

Incorporating Comments on Attachment during Behavioral Parent-Led Play

Goal-directed partnerships have conflict, especially when one of the partners is a toddler or preschooler whose desire to make their own decisions conflicts with their parent's view of reality. After all, why can't a 3-year-old have candy for breakfast, wear shorts in the winter, play with a dead squirrel, or drive a car? Parents have the difficult task of being empathic to their child's desires while enforcing limits needed for their child's safety and healthy development. Behavioral parent-led play provides an opportunity for parents to practice being calmly in charge while remaining empathic to their child's feelings. Examples of coaching statements that reinforce this aspect of healthy parent-child relationships are shown in Table 4.7.

Another aspect of secure attachment relationships that is especially applicable to coaching parent-led play is the concept of "disruption and repair" (Beebe et al. 2010). In secure attachment relationships, there is the expectation there will be efforts to repair the interaction following conflicts or disruptions. Since there is no such expectation in insecure dyads, there is often no resolution to conflicts which makes them seem especially scary. During parent-led play, parents and children have the opportunity to "repair" their relationship through child-led play following conflict. Examples of coaching statements reinforcing the importance of repair following disruption and highlighting the parent and child's efforts at repair are shown in Table 4.8. A form summarizing important principles for coaching parent-led play is shown in Table 4.9.

Table 4.8 Examples of in vivo coaching statements reinforcing repair following disruption

I love the way you go right back to following his lead after he follows directions
That was cool she apologized. She was feeling guilty about tearing up your picture
Child-led play helps children calm down after the time-out. It helps parents and therapists calm down too
Going back to child-led play lets you repair your relationship after the time-out

Table 4.9 Coding parent coaching during parent-led play and discipline

Conveys sense of confidence in parent and discipline process/Calm, decisive demeanor	*Satisfactory*	*Needs practice*
Reminds parent of next steps in discipline process	*Satisfactory*	*Needs practice*
(e.g. "Wait 5 s, one thousand one, one thousand two …; Now give the warning, say "If you don't …)		
Reminds parent of long-term benefits of parent-led play	*Satisfactory*	*Needs practice*
(e.g. "Your home will be calmer when he learns to follow directions.", "It will feel like a safer world to him when he knows you're in charge.")		
Praises parent for positive parenting skills	*Satisfactory*	*Needs practice*
(e.g. "Nice direct command." "Great job of waiting 5 s." "I love the way you pointed when you gave the command." "Nice labeled praise." "I love how calm you are." "Great job of letting him decide whether he is ready to obey.")		
Provides support and distraction for parent during time-out through frequent verbalizations	*Satisfactory*	*Needs practice*
Early parent-led play sessions: Interrupts and corrects problematic commands	*Satisfactory*	*Needs practice*
(e.g. parent says "Can you hand me" and therapist interrupts and says "Say please hand me.")		
Later parent-led play sessions: informs parent when they have given a problematic command		
(e.g. parents says "Can you hand me the blue block?" and therapist says "That was an indirect command.")		
Reminds parent of importance of child-led play/relationship in calming down and reconnecting. Points out importance of repair following time-out	*Satisfactory*	*Needs practice*
(e.g. "Child-led play is so important in helping him calm down after doing something difficult like following directions." "I love how you are focusing on following his lead and not dwelling on the time-out". "That rhythm of working on homework and then playing helps him stay regulated.")		

Conclusions

Whether the theoretical basis for a parent coaching intervention is behaviorism or attachment theory, one of the most important aspects of the coaching is whether the provider's approach to the parent is congruent with the approach they want the parent to use with their child. During parent coaching it is possible to target both improved security of attachment and reduction in behavior problems.

The next four chapters focus on adapting parent coaching to different patterns of attachment/attachment state of mind. Any therapist who has seen more than a handful of families for behavioral parent coaching knows every family and child responds differently. The goal is to give parent coaches a way of thinking about those different responses and tailoring their coaching approach to address them. The advantage of identifying attachment patterns is it will make some of these reactions more predictable and help you understand why the parent and child may react in certain ways at different stages of treatment. Another advantage of identifying pattern of attachment is years of attachment research gives us an idea of how this pattern may have developed (i.e. what child-parent interactions may have looked like when the child was an infant and what the parent's state of mind regarding attachment may be). This can help you be more compassionate with the dyad by understanding why it may be challenging for them to implement specific behavioral strategies. It will also help you to tailor your coaching to the parent's state of mind. Coaching to a parent's attachment state of mind is a balance—you need to be able to see their child and their response from their perspective but, in order for them to respond differently, you need to be careful to not overidentify with their perspective.

Although I am clearly a proponent of using conceptualizations of attachment patterns to guide parent coaching, I also recognize there are potential pitfalls associated with this approach. One potential pitfall is overlooking unique aspects of the child and parent's attachment struggles by reducing them to a category. A related concern is identifying the pattern of attachment may reduce compassion and empathy for the family as therapists begin to think pejoratively about families they struggle with (e.g. "Those parents are so dismissing they will never be able to do child-led play."). In order to guard against these disadvantages, it is important to keep an open mind about how to classify each family's attachment struggles. It is also important interventionists reflect on the types of families they find especially challenging with a colleague, supervisor, or therapist who can provide them with a secure base for exploring their own struggles.

References

Achenbach, T. R. (2000). *Manual for the ASEBA preschool forms & profiles*. Burlington: ASEBA.

Ainsworth, M. (1967). *Infancy in Uganda*. Baltimore: Johns Hopkins Press.

Barnett, M., Niec, L., & Acevedo-Polakovich, I. (2014). Assessing the key to effective coaching in parent-child interaction therapy: The therapist-parent interaction coding system. *Journal of Psychopathology and Behavioral Assessment, 36,* 211–223.

Beebe, B., Jaffe, J., Markese, S., Buck, K., Chen, H., Cohen, P. (2010). The origins of 12-month attachment: A microanalysis of 4-month mother-infant interaction. *Attachment & Human Development, 12*(1), 3–141.

Cassidy, J., Marvin, R., & the MacArthur Working Group on Attachment. (1992). *Attachment organization in preschool children: Procedures and coding guidelines* (4th ed.). Charlottesville: University of Virginia.

Eyberg, S. (2005). Parent-child interaction therapy: Basic coaching guidelines. University of Florida PCIT website: http://pcit.phhp.ufl.edu/…/web%20Coaching%20in%20PCIT%20 May%202006.ppt. Accessed 2 Jan 2014.

Eyberg, S., & Funderburk, B. (2011). *Parent-child interaction therapy protocol*. Gainesville: PCIT International, Inc.

Eyberg, S., & Pincus, D. (1999). *Eyberg child behavior inventory and sutter-eyberg student behavior inventory-revised professional manual*. Lutz: Psychological Assessment Resources, Inc.

Eyberg, S., Nelson, M., Duke, M., & Boggs, S. (2005). Dyadic parent-child interaction coding system (DPICS) (3rd ed.). Accessed 17 Nov 2007.

Eyberg, S., Nelson, M., Ginn, N., Bhuiyan, N., & Boggs, S. (2013). *Dyadic parent-child interaction coding system (DPICS)* (4th ed.). Gainesville: PCIT International, Inc.

Fernandez, M., & Eyberg, S. (2009). Predicting treatment and follow-up attrition in parent-child interaction therapy. *Journal of Abnormal Child Psychology, 37,* 431–441.

Forehand, R., & McMahon, R. (1981). *Helping the noncompliant child: A clinician's guide to parent training*. New York: The Guilford Press.

Herschell, A., Capage, L., Bahl, A., & McNeil, C. (2008). The role of therapist communication style in Parent-Child Interaction Therapy. *Child & Family Behavior Therapy, 30*(1), 13–35.

Hoffman, K., Marvin, R., Cooper, G., & Powell, B. (2006). Changing toddlers' and preschoolers' attachment classifications: The circle of security intervention. *Journal of Consulting and Clinical Psychology, 74,* 1017–1026.

McMahon, C., & Forehand, R. (2003). *Helping the noncompliant child: family-based treatment for oppositional defiant disorder* (2nd ed.). New York: Guilford Press.

McNeil, C., & Hembree-Kigin, T. (2010). *Parent-child interaction therapy* (2nd ed.). New York: Springer.

Main, M., & Goldwyn, R. (1998). *Adult attachment scoring and classification system.* Berkeley: University of California.

Oxford English Dictionary. (Ed.) (2014). Oxford: Oxford University Press.

Patterson, G. (1982). *Coercive family process*. Eugene: Castalia Publishing Company.

Patterson, G., & Forgatch, M. (1985). Therapist behavior as a determinant for client noncompliance: A paradox for the behavior modifier. *Journal of Consulting and Clinical Psychology, 53,* 846–851.

Pawl, J. H., & St. John, M. (1998). How you are is as important as what you do … in making a positive difference for infants, toddlers, and their families. *Zero to Three*.

Pembroke, G. (2014). *Reasons my kid is crying*. Atlanta: Three Rivers Press.

Powell, B., Cooper, G., Hoffman, K., & Marvin, R. (2014). *The circle of security intervention: enhancing attachment in early parent-child relationships*. New York: Guilford.

Siegel, D., & Bryson, T. (2014). 'Time-Outs' are hurting your child. *Time*. http://time.com/3404701/ discipline-time-out-is-not-good/#3404701/discipline-time-out-is-not-good/. Assessed 18 Oct 2014.

Smyke, A., Dumitrescu, A., & Zeanah, C. (2002). Attachment disturbances in young children. *I: The continuum of caretaking casualty, 41*(8), 972–982.

Steele, H., & Steele, M. (2008). *Clinical applications of the adult attachment interview*. New York: Guilford.

Sunderland, M. (2006). *The science of parenting*. London: DK Adult.

Urquiza, A., Zebell, N., McGrath, J., & Whitten, L. (2011). *Course of treatment manual for PCIT-TC*. Davis: University of California at Davis. http://pcit.ucdavis.edu.

van IJzendoorn, M., & Hubbard, F. (2000). Are infant crying and maternal responsiveness during the first year related to infant-mother attachment at 15 months? *Attachment & Human Development, 2*(3), 371–391.

Werba, B., Eyberg, S., Boggs, S., & Algina, J. (2006). Predicting outcome in parent-child interaction therapy. *Behavior Modification, 30*(5), 618–646.

Beth Troutman is a Clinical Professor in Psychiatry at the University of Iowa Carver College of Medicine. Her teaching, research, and clinical work has focused on improving parent-child interactions for more than 30 years. She has had a foot in more than one theoretical camp since graduate school, conducting research on parenting self-efficacy, temperament, and attachment theory and disseminating Parent-Child Interaction Therapy (PCIT), a behavioral model for improving parenting.

Chapter 5
Ordinary Magic

What began as a quest to understand the extraordinary has revealed the power of the ordinary.
(Masten 2001)

Elena[1] *seeks help for herself and her 3 year-old daughter, Penny, due to Penny's noncompliance, arguing, and irritability. During the intake, Elena reports there was a change in her daughter's behavior several months ago. Elena initially attributed the onset of Penny's misbehavior and noncompliance to a combination of the "terrible threes", move to a new community, and birth of a sister. After yelling at Penny one day for coloring on the wall, Elena called a close friend in tears to discuss her concerns about Penny and her reactions to Penny's misbehavior. Her friend reported similar struggles with her son and said they had benefited from an intervention where she was coached while interacting with her son. Elena discussed this option with her husband that evening. Although he felt Penny would outgrow her difficulties, he was sympathetic to his wife's distress and supported her decision to seek help.*

Upon entering the play room for the modified strange situation procedure used to assess child-parent attachment, Penny began exploring the toys in the room, pausing at times to show items to her mother. She was especially excited about her ability to operate the play cash register, delightedly showing her mother how she was able to scan items "just like the grocery store". When the signal was given for Elena to leave the room, she told Penny she had to go to the bathroom and she should stay and play. Elena suggested Penny scan the rest of the grocery items so they could fix dinner when she returned. Penny continued to scan and arrange the grocery items until her mother returned. When Elena returned, Penny turned to greet her when she entered the room saying "Hi, Mom. Let's fix dinner." Elena sat down beside Penny and they pretended to cook dinner until the signal came for

[1] This is a fictional account illustrating characteristics of a secure dyad and a parent with a secure/autonomous state of mind.

B. Troutman, *Integrating Behaviorism and Attachment Theory in Parent Coaching*, SpringerBriefs in Psychology, DOI 10.1007/978-3-319-15239-4_5

Elena to leave again. This time, Penny asked if she could come with her mother. Elena told her she needed to stay in the room and left. Penny looked longingly at the door for several seconds. She then went and gathered blocks, stacked them next to the cash register, and began scanning them. When her mother returned following the separation, Penny ignored her for a few seconds. Her mother said "Are you scanning blocks now?". Penny replied "Yes." She continued scanning blocks and when her mother sat down said, "How many blocks do you want?"

During the child-led portion of the behavioral assessment, Penny and her mother continued to play with the blocks and cash register. They both clearly enjoyed playing together and Elena said "Maybe we should get some blocks like this at home." "And the cash register!" Penny said. When told to switch to parent-led play, Elena moved to a doll house and asked Penny to come play with her. Penny initially refused but her resistance melted when her mother began having the mother and child dolls talk to each other. Penny's mood changed when her mother told her it was time to clean up the toys. After half-heartedly tossing a couple of blocks in the direction of the box, she refused to pick up any more blocks, telling her mother she was "too sad" to clean up.

Overview of Secure Attachment and Secure/Autonomous State of Mind

Hallmarks of secure attachment include clear communication of attachment needs and balance between self- and other-reliance. Anne Masten describes factors associated with resiliency as "ordinary magic" (Masten 2001). One of the handful of factors associated with resiliency is secure attachment. Ordinary magic is an apt description for secure attachment as trainees are sometimes surprised at how perfectly ordinary assessments of securely attached dyads look. The "magic" is in the self-regulation, confidence, and emotional intelligence that comes from the richness of daily experiences providing opportunities for both exploration and attachment.

There are a number of features of the dyad described above (Penny and Elena) that are consistent with secure child-parent attachment and a parent with a secure/autonomous state of mind. The affective sharing and clear communication of feelings, including negative feelings, seen in this dyad is consistent with secure attachment. Another indicator is Penny's balance between exploring the room on her own and seeking reassurance from her mother. Consistent with secure/autonomous state of mind, Elena values her relationship with her daughter and recognizes her role in the conflict that has developed in their interactions. Elena's willingness to seek assistance from others when having difficulties is characteristic of individuals with secure/autonomous state of mind.

Table 5.1 Characteristics of secure infant-parent attachment in the strange situation procedure. (Source: Ainsworth et al. 1978)

Secure (B)	The baby may be distressed during separations from caregiver. If she is distressed, she seeks contact with the parent during the reunions and is easily soothed by the parent. The baby actively seeks interaction with parent after separation with little resistance or avoidance. The baby clearly acknowledges parent's return following separations with smile, cry, or approach. Good quality exploration and play prior to separations and after parent's return
B1	Baby shows little or no distress during separations. He greets the parent upon return and seeks interaction but not physical contact
B2	The baby shows little or no distress during separations. She greets the parent upon return. She may show some initial avoidance of parent following first separation but seek contact with the parent following the second separation
B3	The baby may be distressed during the separation episodes. He actively seeks contact with the parent following separations and will maintain contact by resisting attempts to release him before he is ready. Given his level of distress, his quick recovery following his parent's return is striking
B4	The baby is clearly distressed during separations, especially during the second separation where he seems entirely distressed. He seeks contact with the parent and, although there may be some evidence of mixed feelings, he clearly seeks to maintain contact with his parent

Characteristics of Secure Attachment

Characteristics of securely attached dyads in research-based observational assessments of attachment (strange situation procedure and modified strange situation procedure for preschool children) are summarized in Tables 5.1 and 5.2. Securely attached infants (aged 12–18 months) often exhibit distress when separated from the parent. Regardless of whether he is distressed during the separation, a securely attached infant will seek contact with his parent when he returns following a brief separation. If the infant is distressed, he calms quickly when his parent returns and soon returns to exploration. The increase in cognitive and verbal skills from infancy to early childhood impacts how securely attached preschoolers (2½–4½) respond to separation and reunion. Securely attached preschool-aged children rarely exhibit significant distress at separation although they may negotiate with their parent not to leave or exhibit muted exploration and play while the parent is gone. The reaction of securely attached preschoolers to the parent's return also seems less dramatic than the securely attached infant's response to reunion. The interactions of securely attached preschoolers and their parents are marked by calm, comfortable enjoyment of interacting with each other both before and after the separation.

Table 5.2 Characteristics of secure child-parent attachment in modified separation-reunion procedure for preschool children. (Source: Cassidy and Marvin 1992)

Secure (B)	Child is interested in interacting with the parent. Child rarely shows extensive crying during separation but may exhibit muted exploration or search for parent. Child may exhibit no distress during separation—continuing to play until parent returns. Child displays relaxed pleasure at parent's return. Following parent's return, interaction picks up where it left off prior to separation
Secure-reserved (B1)	Child displays some initial avoidance or reserve following separation. However, after a relatively short period of time (a minute or less) engages in happy, intimate interaction with parent
Very secure (B3)	Child clearly enjoys interacting with the parent. Interactions appear calm and comfortable with almost no avoidance, ambivalence, disorganized, or controlling behavior
Secure-dependent (B4)	Child displays some initial pouty or immature behavior following separation communicating hurt feelings or displeasure in the context of generally secure behavior
Secure-feisty (B4)	Child is confidently assertive in interactions with parent. Child seems interested in showing off for parent, emphasizing both the relationship and their ability to make their own choices
Secure-controlling (B4)	Child's interactions with parent are generally secure with one or two isolated instances of trying to control parent
Secure-other (B other)	Child clearly uses parent as secure base and safe haven but does not clearly fall into specific subgroup

Rates of Secure Attachment

As early interventionists focused on improving parent-child interactions, it is easy to become focused on what is not working in the relationship. It is reassuring to remember most children have a secure attachment relationship with at least one parent (54–78 % in community samples) (Greenberg et al. 1991; Kochanska and Kim 2013; Leigh et al. 2004; Moss et al. 2004; Speltz et al. 1990, 1999; Troutman et al. 2010; van Ijzendoorn et al. 1999) and 40 % are securely attached to both parents (Kochanska and Kim 2013).

Although secure attachment is a protective factor, it is not a guarantee against conflicts in the parent-child relationship, including conflicts significant enough for the child to meet criteria for a disruptive behavior disorder. In clinical samples, the rate of secure attachment is significantly lower than community samples but one-fifth to one-third of dyads referred for clinical services are securely attached (Cohen et al. 1999; Greenberg et al. 1991; Speltz et al. 1990, 1995). The lowest rate of secure attachment is seen in families where a child has experienced physical abuse, neglect, or sexual abuse (3–25 %) (Cicchetti et al. 2006; Moss et al. 2011).

Table 5.3 Characteristics of secure/autonomous attachment state of mind in Adult Attachment Interview (AAI). (Source: Main and Goldwyn 1998)

Secure/Autonomous (F)	Values attachment relationships and experiences. Generalized descriptions of relationships with parents (semantic level) are supported by specific memories. Adult either supports descriptions of parents as loving during childhood or reflects on parents' lack of loving behavior without angry preoccupation or idealization (earned secure)
Some setting aside of attachment (F1)	Mild, unexamined sense of support from parents or describes conscious decision to not dwell on negative aspects of caregiving
Some detachment (F2)	Similar to F3 but some indices of detachment such as difficulty supporting positive statements about parenting due to lack of memory or idealization of parents. May describe some mild derogation of parents mixed with overall valuing of attachment
Very secure (F3)	Descriptions of parenting at the semantic level are supported by specific memories. Descriptions are fresh, coherent, and contained whether childhood experiences were easy or difficult
Slightly preoccupied (F4)	Somewhat sentimental about supportive childhood or slightly confused by traumatic experiences
Somewhat resentful/conflicted (F5)	Somewhat preoccupied with problematic parenting but anger is contained or accompanied by humor. Accepting of flawed relationship

Parenting Behaviors Associated with Secure Attachment

As described in Chap. 2, parenting behaviors associated with the development of secure attachment include sensitive responsiveness to attachment cues (especially distress cues), support for exploration, affective attunement, delight in the child, and physical contact, especially in response to distress.

Secure/Autonomous State of Mind

The parental attachment state of mind associated with secure attachment is secure/autonomous. Individuals with a secure/autonomous state of mind tell the story of their childhood in a fresh manner—i.e. as though they are thoughtfully choosing their words. They indicate they value attachment relationships and experiences. The story is internally consistent regardless of whether they describe a loving or harsh childhood. The range of characteristics of Adult Attachment Interview (AAI) transcripts are shown in Table 5.3.

Rates of secure/autonomous state of mind are similar to rates of secure infant and toddler attachment with approximately half of adolescents and adults in community samples (48–59 %) classified with secure/autonomous state of mind using the Adult Attachment Interview (AAI) (Booth-LaForce and Roisman 2014; Caspers et al. 2007; Van Ijzendoorn 1995; van IJzendoorn and Bakermans-Kranenburg 2008).

Similar rates of secure/autonomous state of mind (47–57 %) are seen in low-income mothers participating in a study of an attachment-based home visiting intervention (Korfmacher et al. 1997). Among parents of infants with secure infant-parent attachment, the vast majority (73 %) are classified with secure/autonomous attachment state of mind (Van Ijzendoorn 1995). Rates of secure/autonomous attachment are lower among mothers seeking treatment for their child's conduct problems (22 %) (Routh et al. 1995) and patients participating in psychotherapy outcome studies (5–30 %) (Levy et al. 2006; Stovall-McClough and Cloitre 2003; Talia et al. 2014).

Research on Secure/Autonomous State of Mind

In a small study examining behavioral and neural responses to infant crying, women with secure/autonomous state of mind exhibit less amygdala hyperactivity on functional Magnetic Resonance Imaging when listening to infant crying than women with insecure states of mind (dismissing, preoccupied, and unresolved) (Riem et al. 2012) indicating infant crying is less anxiety-provoking and aversive for secure/autonomous women. Women with secure/autonomous states of mind also rate infant crying as less irritating and are less likely to respond to crying with excessive force (as assessed with handgrip dynamometer) (Riem et al. 2012). Physiological measures of mother's responses to infant distress also indicate mothers with secure/autonomous state of mind find crying less aversive (Ablow et al. 2013).

Secure/autonomous mothers are described by interventionists providing an attachment-based parenting intervention as more emotionally committed to the intervention than mothers with insecure (dismissing or unresolved) states of mind (interventionists were not informed of mothers' state of mind) (Korfmacher et al. 1997). Consistent with the goals of the intervention, secure/autonomous mothers seek assistance with parenting tasks (69 %) and rarely seek crisis intervention (3 %) (Korfmacher et al. 1997). Behavioral observations of psychotherapy sessions find individuals with secure/autonomous state of mind are more likely to express distress, ask for help, and express gratitude than individuals with an insecure state of mind (Talia et al. 2014).

Clinical Observations and Recommendations

Parents with secure/autonomous state of mind are considered good candidates for behavioral parent-child interventions as "unencumbered by preoccupation, disorientation, or denial of the importance of past relationships, are better able to learn and use the "here-and-now" skills important to current relationships" (Greenberg et al. 1991). When coaching parents with autonomous/secure state of mind, it is a joy to see ordinary magic at work. I find these parents "psychologically sturdy". They are open to learning new ways to manage their child's behavior and able to look at their contribution to negative interactions with their child. They are able to forgive themselves for past parenting "mistakes" and to change their parenting approach without excessive guilt or blame. Due to this openness, it is possible to give parents with an autonomous/secure state of mind corrective feedback without meeting with resistance. However, since parents in securely attached dyads tend to be less critical of their children, it is also much easier to get into the positive reinforcement cycle described earlier.

In dyads where the child is securely attached to at least one parent, I find the child tends to give both parents the benefit of the doubt. There may be mild resistance to the parents' efforts to change their patterns of interacting with the child but it tends not to persist.

In my clinical experience, the positive response to behavioral child-led play is often amazingly quick in securely attached dyads—much quicker than I am able to explain based solely on behavioral principles. I think this has something to do with a phenomenon known as security priming (Mikulincer and Shaver 2001). There is a large body of research in adults using experimental manipulations suggesting the availability of attachment figures (e.g. Picasso drawing of mother cradling an infant, guided imagery concerning availability of attachment figures). This research literature finds brief security priming manipulations have positive effects on mood, prosocial feelings, and prosocial behavior (Cassidy and Shaver 2008). For adults with autonomous/secure state of mind, what better security priming technique than spending five minutes of quality time with your child? I think this positive interaction with their child reminds them of their own positive experiences with caregivers, activates their caregiving system, and helps them remember what they cherish about their child.

Priming effects have been found in children as young as 18 months (Over and Carpenter 2009). In this study, young children were shown a photograph prime for affiliation or independence. Children shown a photograph prime for affiliation were three times more likely to spontaneously help an adult than those shown a neutral or independence prime. For children with a secure attachment relationship with their caregivers, I think five minutes a day where their caregiver is following their lead is a powerful affiliation prime that promotes prosocial behavior and motivation to please their caregiver.

Parents with secure/autonomous state of mind express concern about ignoring their child's attachment signals during time-out. They are sensitive to indicators of their child's distress, e.g. crying and indicators of positive attachment signals e.g. saying "I love you Mommy." or "I need a hug.". These are often the most difficult aspects for therapists (and the therapists in nearby offices) to hear as well. When coaching parents through these difficult discipline moments, it is important to acknowledge the real distress experienced by the child and parent. In order to help parents empathize with their child's struggles during these difficult moments, it is important for us to empathize with the parents' struggles. Although it can be tempting to discount the child's statements as manipulative or focus on how the child's behavior or choice led him to be in time-out, it is more helpful to acknowledge the true distress the child is experiencing. However, it is also important to remind parents of the positive long-term consequences for children of learning to follow directions and accept limits—the reason for putting them, their child, and us through this distress. After the child has taken the time-out and returned to positive interactions with the parent, the coach needs to help the parent see the child's ability to calm and return to positive interactions.

Conclusions

Parent coaching is often highly effective at reducing conflict and disruptive behavior in dyads with secure attachment and secure/autonomous state of mind. By reinforcing healthy patterns of behavior, child-led play helps the parent and child build on the healthy foundation in place. As they develop a more enjoyable relationship, there is often a reduction in conflict and negative interactions. Parent-led play and discipline provides parents with the tools to increase compliance and address behavior problems. This helps reduce conflict between the parent and child and improves the parent's sense of competence in managing difficult situations with their child.

References

Ablow, J., Marks, A., Feldman, S., & Huffman, L. (2013). Associations between first-tie expectant women's representations of attachment and their physiological reactivity to infant cry. *Child Development, 84,* 1373–1391.

Ainsworth, M., Blehar, M., Waters, E., & Wall, S. (1978). *Patterns of attachment: A psychological study of the strange situation.* Hillsdale: Erlbaum.

Booth-LaForce, C., & Roisman, G. (2014). The adult attachment interview: Psychometrics, stability and change from infancy, and develpmental origins. *Monographs of the Society for Research in Child Development, 79*(3), 1–185.

Caspers, K., Yucuis, R., Troutman, B., Arndt, S., & Langbehn, D. (2007). A sibling adoption study of adult attachment: The influence of shared environment on attachment state of mind. *Attachment & Human Development, 9*(4), 375–391.

Cassidy, J., & Marvin, R. (1992). *Attachment organization in three and four year olds: Procedures and coding manual.* Charlottesville: University of Virginia.

Cassidy, J., & Shaver, P. (Eds.). (2008). *Handbook of attachment* (2nd ed.). New York: Guilford Press.

Cicchetti, D., Rogosch, F., & Toth, S. (2006). Fostering secure attachment in infants in maltreating families through preventive interventions. *Development and Psychopathology, 18,* 623–649.

Cohen, N., Muir, E., Lojkasek, M., Muir, R., Parker, C., Barwick, M., & Brown, M. (1999). Watch, wait and wonder: Testing the effectiveness of a new approahc to mother-infant psychotherapy. *Infant Mental Health Journal, 20,* 429–451.

Greenberg, M., Speltz, M., DeKlyen, M., & Endriga, M. (1991). Attachment security in preschoolers with and without externalizing behavior problems: A replication. *Development and Psychopathology, 3,* 413–430.

Kochanska, G., & Kim, S. (2013). Early attachment organization with both parents and future behavior problems: From infancy to middle childhood. *Child Development, 84*(1), 283–296.

Korfmacher, J., Adam, E., Ogawa, J., & Egeland, B. (1997). Adult attachment: Implications for the therapeutic process in a home visitation intervention. *Applied Developmental Science, 1*(1), 43–52.

Leigh, I., Brice, P., & Meadow-Orlans, K. (2004). Attachment in deaf mothers and their children. *Journal of Deaf Studies and Deaf Education, 9*(2), 176–188.

Levy, K., Meehan, K., Kelly, K., Reynoso, J., Weber, M., Clarkin, J., & Kernberg, O. (2006). Change in attachment patterns and reflective function in a randomized control trial of transference-focused psychotherapy for borderline personality disorder. *Journal of Consulting and Clinical Psychology, 74*(6), 1027–1040.

Main, M., & Goldwyn, R. (1998). *Adult attachment scoring and classification system*. Berkeley: University of California.

Masten, A. (2001). Ordinary magic. Resilience processes in development. *American Psychologist, 56*(3), 227–238.

Mikulincer, M., & Shaver, P. (2001). Attachment theory and intergroup bias: Evidence that priming the secure base schema attenuates negative reactions to out-groups. *Journal of Personality and Social Psychology, 81,* 97–115.

Moss, E., Cyr, C., & Dubois-Comtois, K. (2004). Attachment at early school age and developmental risk: Examining family contexts and behavior problems of controlling-caregiving, controlling-punitive, and behaviorally disorganized children. *Developmental Psychology, 40*(4), 519–532.

Moss, E., Dubois-Comtois, K., Cyr, C., St-Laurent, D., & Bernier, A. (2011). Efficacy of a home-visiting intervention aimed at improving maternal sensitivity, child attachment, and behavioral outcomes for maltreated children: A randomized control trial. *Development and Psychopathology, 23,* 195–210.

Over, H., & Carpenter, M. (2009). Eighteenth-month-old infants show increased helping following priming with affiliation. *Psychological Science, 20*(10), 1189–1193.

Riem, M., Bakermans-Kranenburg, M., van Ijzendoorn, M., Out, D., & Rombouts, S. (2012). Attachment in the brain: adult attachment representations predict amygdala and behavioral responses to infant crying. *Attachment & Human Development, 14*(6), 533–551.

Routh, C., Hill, J., Steele, H., Elliott, C., & Dewey, M. (1995). Maternal attachment status, psychosocial stressors and problem behaviour: Follow-up after parent training courses for conduct disorder. *Journal of Child Psychology and Psychiatry, 36*(7), 1179–1198.

Speltz, M., Greenberg, M., & DeKlyen, M. (1990). Attachment in preschoolers with disruptive behavior: A comparison of clinic-referred and nonproblem children. *Development and Psychopathology, 2,* 31–46.

Speltz, M., DeKlyen, M., Greenberg, M., & Dryden, M. (1995). Clinic referral for oppositional defiant disorder: Relative significance of attachment and behavioral variables. *Journal of Abnormal Child Psychology, 23*(4), 487–507.

Speltz, M., DeKlyen, M., & Greenberg, M. (1999). Attachment in boys with early onset conduct problems. *Development and Psychopathology, 11,* 269–285.

Stovall-McClough, K., & Cloitre, M. (2003). Reorganization of unresolved childhood traumatic memories following exposure therapy. *Annals of the New York Academy of Sciences, 2008,* 297–299.

Talia, A., Daniel, S., Miller-Bottome, M., Brambilla, D., Miccoli, D., Safran, J., & Lingiardi, V. (2014). AAI predicts patients' in-session interpersonal behavior and discourse: A "move to the level of the relation" for attachment-informed psychotherapy research. *Attachment & Human Development, 16*(2), 192–209.

Troutman, B., Arndt, S., Caspers, K., & Yucuis, R. (2010). *Infant negative emotionality moderates the association between quantity of nonfamilial day care and infant-mother attachment.* Paper presented at the scientific proceedings of the American academy of child & adolescent psychiatry's 57th annual meeting, New York.

Van Ijzendoorn, M. (1995). Adult attachment representations, parental responsiveness, and infant attachment: A meta-analysis on the predictive validity of the adult attachment interview. *Psychological Bulletin, 117*(3), 387–403.

van IJzendoorn, M., & Bakermans-Kranenburg, M. (2008). The distribution of adult attachment representations in clinical groups: A meta-analytic search for patterns of attachment in 105 AAI studies. In H. Steele & M. Steele (Eds.), *Clinical applications of the adult attachment interview*. New York: Guilford Press.

van Ijzendoorn, M., Schuengel, C., & Bakermans-Kranenberg, M. (1999). Disorganized attachment in early childhood: Meta-analysis of precursors, concomitants, and sequelae. *Development and Psychopathology, 11*, 225–249.

Beth Troutman PhD is a Clinical Professor in Psychiatry at the University of Iowa Carver College of Medicine. Her teaching, research, and clinical work has focused on improving parent-child interactions for more than 30 years. She has had a foot in more than one theoretical camp since graduate school, conducting research on parenting self-efficacy, temperament, and attachment theory and disseminating Parent-Child Interaction Therapy (PCIT), a behavioral model for improving parenting.

Chapter 6
Can't Live With Her, Can't Live Without Her

As you move in, I move away; as I move away, you move in...No matter where I move in relation to you, I cannot get comfortable.
(Beebe et al. 2010)

Three-year-old Janey was referred by her pediatrician following a recent, especially trying well child visit[1]*. The primary concerns of Janey's pediatrician include separation anxiety, oppositional behavior, and aggression. Janey's aggression is often directed towards her mother. Janey attends preschool two mornings a week. During the intake interview, Janey's mother, Callie, says she is considering taking Janey out of preschool due to the difficulty in getting Janey to separate. Callie indicates she is interested in learning more effective discipline techniques as Janey "runs all over her" and "fails to listen to her". Callie tearfully describes her own mother as a harsh disciplinarian and adamantly states she does not want to repeat that pattern with her daughter. When asked about her support system, Callie describes her mother as her best friend and says she talks to her every day. Callie is divorced and Janey spends every other weekend with her father. Callie speaks angrily of her ex-husband and describes Janey as an "emotional mess" when she returns from visits with her father.*

After entering the play room with her mother, Janey begins to pull on her mother's arm and whine for her mother to play with her. When her mother sits on the floor to play with her, Janey begins trying to build a tower out of blocks. When the tower falls down, Janey asks her mother to build a tower for her whining "I can't do it". When the signal comes for Janey's mother to leave the room, she gets up and tells Janey she is leaving. When asked why, Janey's mother states "because the doctor told me I have to leave". This leads into an extended discussion between Janey and her mother with Janey questioning why she cannot go with her mother.

[1] This is a fictional account illustrating characteristics of an ambivalent/resistant dyad and a parent with a preoccupied state of mind.

B. Troutman, *Integrating Behaviorism and Attachment Theory in Parent Coaching*, SpringerBriefs in Psychology, DOI 10.1007/978-3-319-15239-4_6

After her mother leaves, Janey stands at the door and cries. Her mother is sent back in the room in 30 s due to Janey's distress. When her mother enters the room, Janey begins angrily asking her why she left her by herself. Her mother attempts to explain this to her but Janey becomes more and more angry, yelling at her mother and hitting her. When the signal comes for the second separation, Janey hangs on her mother as she attempts to leave. Janey again stands crying at the door during the separation. When her mother returns, she immediately begins arguing with her mother. They continue to argue throughout the reunion and Janey does not return to exploration of the toys.

During observations of child-led play and parent-led play, Janey becomes increasingly frustrated and whiny as her mother attempts to engage her in the play with questions and indirect commands. When Janey's mother tentatively asks her if she wants to pick up the toys, Janey bursts into tears stating "it's not fair" she has to clean up since her mother also played with the toys.

Overview of Ambivalent/Resistant Attachment and Preoccupied State of Mind

Ambivalent/resistant attachment is characterized by a combination of distress when the parent is absent but inability to be comforted when the parent is present. The term ambivalent refers to the apparent paradox presented by the child exhibiting separation distress when the mother leaves but not being comforted when the parent returns. The term resistant refers to the child resisting contact with the mother (either active resistance such as pushing away from the mother or hitting the mother or passive resistance such as not seeking comfort/not being soothed). Children in these dyads tend to be clingy and highly focused on the attachment relationship with limited exploration. This has been described as hyperactivation of the attachment system.

Presenting problems often include both separation anxiety and disruptive behavior. There may also be aggression directed towards the parent. During child-led play, there tends to be a pattern of "pursue and retreat" with the parent pursuing and trying to entice the child into playing with her and the child withdrawing from the parent's initiatives. Children in these dyads may also reject overtures for physical contact by the parent such as rubbing the child's back or trying to cuddle or hug the child. From the parent's perspective, she feels constantly rejected by the child which heightens her need to pursue the child. From the child's perspective, the parent's overtures are intrusive and not in response to her attachment needs so she tends to protect herself by withdrawing. However, when the parent leaves or indicates she is going to leave, the child's attachment needs are heightened. Since the child perceives the parent as unpredictable, she does not feel confident the parent will return, leading to separation distress. The child's dilemma regarding their parent is "can't live with her and can't live without her". So, she is vigilant about her parent's whereabouts but does not enjoy or feel relaxed in interactions with her parents.

Table 6.1 Description of ambivalent/resistant attachment in infant-caregiver dyads. (Source: Ainsworth et al. 1978)

Ambivalent/ resistant (C)	The baby is distressed during separations. During the reunions, the baby both resists and seeks contact with the caregiver
C1	The baby is extremely distressed during separations. During reunions, resistant behavior (mixed with contact seeking) is especially notable. There is an angry quality to the interaction
C2	The baby appears passive both in limited exploratory behavior and failure to actively initiate interactions with caregiver. During reunions, the baby signals need for contact but resists contact

Table 6.2 Description of ambivalent/resistant attachment in preschool child-caregiver dyads. (Source: Cassidy and Marvin 1992)

Ambivalent (C)	The child seems reluctant to explore and preoccupied with parent. However, interactions are not relaxed and child seems unable to be comforted by parent. The child may try to involve the parent in interaction by stating he can't do something but then protest or resist parent's attempts to interact. Child protests separation from parent and may be highly distressed or angry during separation. During the reunions, the child appears angry and frustrated, continuing to alternatively seek and reject contact
Resistant (C1)	Parent-child struggle is prominent. This may involve child wanting to engage in some activity while the parent actively discourages the activity or the child resisting the parent's involvement in play. Struggle may escalate to the point of child hitting the parent
Immature (C2)	The child appears immature, seeking the parent's attention through baby talk, clinging, or following parent. The child is unable to use the parent as a secure base for exploration. The child is preoccupied with the parent but does not seem to enjoy interactions with the parent

Research on Ambivalent/Resistant Attachment

Characteristics of ambivalent/resistant attachment are summarized in Tables 6.1 and 6.2. Approximately 10% of community samples of infants and preschool-aged children exhibit ambivalent/resistant attachment with caregivers (Booth-LaForce and Roisman 2014; Kochanska and Kim 2013; Moss et al. 2004; van Ijzendoorn et al. 1999). A similar rate is found in preschool-aged children referred for disruptive behavior (Greenberg et al. 1991; Speltz et al. 1990, 1999).

Research on Parenting Behaviors Associated with Ambivalent/Resistant Attachment

Caregivers in dyads with this pattern of attachment tend to respond inconsistently to their child's attachment needs. Longer work hours, parenting stress, and placement in group day care have also been associated with ambivalent infant-mother attachment (Scher and Mayseless 2000). Mothers in dyads with ambivalent attachment report more separation anxiety than mothers of securely attached dyads (Scher and Mayseless 2000). Dyads with ambivalent/resistant attachment at 15 months have significantly more episodes of a pattern described as "chase and dodge" during face-to-face interactions at four months of age (Beebe et al. 2010). That is, when the infant looked away from the mother to modulate arousal, the mother would "chase" the child to make eye contact by moving her head towards the infant's face. Mothers of infants who develop ambivalent/resistant attachment use more intrusive touch (scratching, pulling, pushing, poking, pinching) with their infants and, by four months of age, their infants are not emotionally organized by their mother's touch (Beebe et al. 2010). Thus, while physical contact typically contributes to the development of a secure attachment, for young children who have experienced excessive intrusive touch from their caregivers, physical contact with their caregiver may be dysregulating. Infants with an ambivalent/resistant attachment with their caregiver cannot count on their caregiver's availability so need to maintain constant vigilance rather than exploring. However, they are also on guard against intrusive interactions with their caregiver so are unable to relax and accept comfort from her when she is available.

It has been hypothesized that inconsistent responding in some caregivers in ambivalent/resistant dyads may result from an unconscious desire to heighten the child's attachment behavior (Beebe et al. 2010). In other caregivers, the inconsistent responding may be the result of parenting stress (Scher and Mayseless 2000).

Outcome Studies on Attachment-Based Interventions: Rate of Ambivalent/Resistant Attachment

As shown in Tables 6.3 and 6.4, the relatively low rates of ambivalent/resistant attachment make conclusions about which attachment-based interventions are especially effective at reducing ambivalent/resistant attachment tentative. However, a variety of approaches focusing on providing parents with support and increasing parents' sensitive responsiveness to attachment signals seem to be associated with reductions in ambivalent/resistant attachment. In families with a history of maltreatment, interventions that provide support to parents and reinforce maternal sensitive responsiveness are associated with improvements in ambivalent/resistant attachment (Cicchetti et al. 2006; Moss et al. 2011). In dyads with irritable infants, a skills-based intervention focused on improving sensitive responsiveness (van den Boom 1994) is associated with improvement in ambivalent/resistant attachment while the Circle of Security home visiting approach (Cassidy et al. 2011) is not. One of the strategies used for intrusive mother of irritable babies in van den Boom's (1994) approach is having the mother describe what her infant is doing which may reduce the pattern of chase and dodge reported in ambivalent/resistant dyads. The Circle of Security (COS) protocol used in an at-risk Head Start group also fails to lead to a decrease in the rate of ambivalent/resistant attachment (Hoffman et al. 2006).

Table 6.3 Ambivalent/resistant attachment outcomes in intervention studies

Population	Model	Rate of ambivalent/ resistant attachment	Reference
Infants in maltreating families (United States) N=137	Child-parent psychotherapy (CPP)	Pre CPP: 3%	(Cicchetti et al. 2006)
		Post CPP: 0%	
	Nurse family partnership (NFP)	Pre NFP: 4%	
		Post NFP: 0%	
	Community standard care (CS)	Pre CS: 4%	
		Post CS: 2%	
Toddlers of mothers with Postpartum Major depressive disorder (United States) N=130	Child-parent psychotherapy (CPP)	Pre CPP: 9%	(Toth et al. 2006)
		Post CPP: 4%	
	Control (Con)	Pre Con: 9%	
		Post Con: 7%	
At-risk head start and early head start group (United States) N=65	Circle of security (COS)	Pre COS: 3%	(Hoffman et al. 2006)
		Post COS: 11%	
First born, irritable infants in economically stressed households (United States) N=220	Circle of security—home visiting-4 intervention (COS-HV4)	COS-HV4: 15%	(Cassidy et al. 2011)
	Control (Con)	Con: 15%	

Table 6.4 Ambivalent/resistant attachment outcomes in parent coaching interventions

Population	Model	Rate of ambivalent/ resistant attachment	Reference
First born, irritable infants in low socio-economic households (Netherlands) N=100 @ 12 mos.; 82 @ 18 mos	Skills-based intervention (SBI) control (Con)	SBI @ 12 mos.: 6% SBI @ 18 mos.: 2% Con @ 12 mos.: 14% Con @ 18 mos.: 13%	(van den Boom 1994)
Maltreated infants and preschool-aged children (Canada) N=67	Relationship intervention program (RIP) community services (CS)	Pre RIP: 6% Post RIP: 0% Pre CS: 16% Post CS: 9%	(Moss et al. 2011)

Characteristics of Preoccupied State of Mind

Characteristics of preoccupied state of mind are summarized in Table 6.5. Preoccupied state of mind occurs in 3–10% of adolescents and adults (Bakermans-Kranenburg et al. 2009; Booth-LaForce and Roisman 2014; Caspers et al. 2007). Rates are also relatively low in parents seeking help with parenting (1–5%) (Korfmacher et al. 1997; Routh et al. 1995). Rates are somewhat higher among patients receiving psychotherapy for borderline personality disorder (15%) (Levy et al. 2006).

Table 6.5 Description of preoccupied state of mind in adult attachment interview (AAI). (Main and Goldwyn 1998)

Preoccupied/entangled (E)	Preoccupied with early attachment experiences. Neither dismisses nor coherently describes caregiving. Vacillates between positive and negative evaluations of parents
Passive (E1)	Impression of excessive involvement in family relationships. Positive view of childhood but sense of letting the parents down
Angry/conflicted (E2)	Extensive discussion of past and current difficulties in relationships
Fearfully preoccupied by traumatic events (E3)	Seems confused, fearful, and overwhelmed by frightening attachment experiences. References to traumatic experiences repeatedly invade speech

Research on Preoccupied State of Mind

In face-to-face interactions with their infant at six months of age, mothers who are more preoccupied tend to become intrusive if their infant is not distressed but to withdraw if their infant is distressed (Haltigan et al. 2014). This is similar to the "chase and dodge" pattern described by Beebe in dyads who develop an ambivalent pattern of attachment. It suggests parents with a preoccupied state of mind have a pattern of responding to their child's distress that keeps the child focused on the attachment relationship and negative emotions as the focus of the relationship.

In individual therapy, individuals with a preoccupied state of mind tend to seek help from the therapist but also resist the therapist's help (Talia et al. 2014). They may "enlist" the opinions of others and quote them to the therapist to support their point of view (Talia et al. 2014). Similar to the pattern of attachment with their child, there seems to be a tendency to keep therapy focused on negative emotions and problems.

Clinical Observations and Recommendations

Countertransference Reactions

When coaching parents with insecure states of mind, the most important work I do is the internal work related to my countertransference reactions. When I am able to use my countertransference reactions to understand the parent and child's experience and develop a collaborative relationship, my coaching flows in a way that is similar to my coaching of securely attached dyads. Just as research on parents' attachment state of mind and infant-parent attachment indicates a "gap" in the specific behaviors that link state of mind and attachment, I am often unaware of the specific ways in which addressing my personal feelings and beliefs about a family affects my interactions with them.

In working with dyads with an ambivalent/resistant attachment relationship, the central concept to remember is hyperactivation of attachment signals. Given this hyperactivation, it is not surprising that observing and coaching these dyads leads to strong emotional reactions from providers. However, the intensity of the reactions and how we manage the reactions varies depending on our own state of mind. Many individuals view the tendency of children in these dyads to seem angry or overwhelmed by distress during separations but to resist their caregiver's attempts to soothe them when they return with irritation. Some interventionists find they feel angry at the child for seeming so "spoiled" and some find they feel angry at the mother for her incompetence. When observing infant strange situation procedures, some individuals are angry with the stranger due to her inability to soothe the child during the separations. Other providers respond to these dyads with sadness at the painful dance between the baby and caregiver and a sense of hopelessness at being able to effect change in their pattern of interactions. The behavioral response to the feelings evoked by these dyads also varies but it often involves rescuing someone. Some interventionists feel a pull to rescue the parents from the child, other people, or life circumstances. For these therapists, the risk is spending too much time at the beginning of in vivo coaching sessions on the parent's problems or identifying too strongly with the parent's view of the child as unmanageable.

Other providers will feel a pull to rescue the child from their parent's incompetence. For these therapists, the pull is to intervene themselves during the session (e.g. by entering the session and stopping the play when the child becomes aggressive rather than having the parent end the play) or by switching to a different approach such as individual play therapy in order to provide the child with a competent surrogate parent.

The tendency of individuals with a preoccupied state of mind to wallow in problems and negative emotions often leads me to feel stuck when working with these dyads. Like quicksand, it feels like the more I struggle to convince the parent their interactions with their child can be different or to try to get them to change their pattern of interaction, the more stuck I feel. I have learned the importance of making observations that help the parent see their emerging capacities. I have also learned that given the parent's overlearned tendency to get their attachment needs met by telling providers the worst, they often need ongoing support for competence from me long after they demonstrate improved interactions with their child.

Coaching Child-Led Play

In order for the child to relax and enjoy child-led play with the parent, the parent needs to quit pursuing the child and let the child come to them. I believe the term "Parent-Child Interaction Therapy" evokes the preoccupied parent's model of their ideal parent-child relationship—one in which their child is completely responsive to their needs for attention and affection. Thus, the child-led play part of this behavioral parenting intervention may heighten the parent's anxiety and need for their child to interact with them. I address this by telling the parent that although the therapy is called Parent-Child Interaction Therapy that does not necessarily mean their child will always be interacting with them. I explain that part of typical development/healthy attachment at this age is the child learning to go off and do activities by themselves. When the parent is able to do this, the child will eventually seek interactions with the parent which reduces the parent's anxiety about being rejected. Once the parent gives the child some space to engage in their own activities, the child will typically begin to give nonverbal indications of wanting to interact with the parent (e.g. glancing at the parent, coming to the parent to show them something, or coming over to see what the parent is doing). The parent can then begin following the child's lead.

Parents in these dyads typically struggle with setting limits and being an authority figure for their child. Their model of relationships is that the child should want to please them so they should not need to set limits. Given this struggle, the end of child-led play coaching sessions is typically difficult. I try to begin shaping a better end to the session by having the parent give the child a warning that play time is almost over 2–5 min before the end of the session. If the child "accepts" this (I basically count just about anything other than throwing a big tantrum as accepting), I then have the parent praise the child for accepting that special play is almost over. Children can be given multiple warnings (e.g. 10 min left, 5 min left, 2 min left) to create several opportunities for accepting the end of the session.

Coaching Parent-Led Play and Discipline

Parents with a more preoccupied state of mind are concerned that setting limits, giving their child commands, and disciplining their child are likely to harm their attachment relationship. Parents in these dyads are often reluctant to give direct commands or use time-out from positive reinforcement, especially since there is often significant improvement in their child's behavior with the implementation of child-led play.

When talking with parents about parent-led play, I find it helpful to describe this as the next step in improving their relationship with their child, emphasizing that it is important to their child's safety for them to be calmly in charge. When parents in these dyads need to set a limit with their child, they tend to be very indirect about expectations such as saying "Do we need to take a time-out?" If they try to give their child a time-out, they tend to hover over the chair or cuddle the child on the chair which contributes to increased conflict and both the parent and child becoming increasingly dysregulated and upset.

I view parent-led play as an opportunity to continue the work begun during child-led play coaching sessions in helping the parent allow the child more autonomy. The parent gives the child clear commands and clearly states the consequences for noncompliance but must let the child choose how to respond. Given these dyads long-standing history of conflict, it is important for both the parent and child to have the experience of child-led play after the child has followed a command or taken a time-out. They begin to get the sense of the rhythm of healthy relationships where there can be periods of conflict followed by periods of enjoyable interactions.

Conclusions

Effective parent coaching with dyads with ambivalent/resistant attachment and parents with preoccupied state of mind involves helping dyads quit chasing and dodging each other so the time they spend together is less conflictual and more enjoyable. Providers can use child-led play to help parents learn to provide more scaffolding of their child's exploration. Parent-led play can be used to help parents learn to provide the hierarchical parent-child relationship needed for children to be safe and thrive.

References

Ainsworth, M., Blehar, M., Waters, E., & Wall, S. (1978). *Patterns of attachment: A psychological study of the strange situation*. Hillsdale: Erlbaum.

Bakermans-Kranenburg, M., & van IJzendoorn, M. (2009). The first 10,000 adult attachment interviews: Distributions of adult attachment representations in clinical and non-clinical groups. *Attachment & Human Development, 11*(3), 223–263.

Beebe, B., Jaffe, J., Markese, S., Buck, K., Chen, H., Cohen, P., Feldstein, S., et al. (2010). The origins of 12-month attachment: A microanalysis of 4 month mother-infant interaction. *Attachment & Human Development, 12*(1), 3–141.

Booth-LaForce, C., & Roisman, G. (2014). The adult attachment interview: Psychometrics, stability and change from infancy, and develpmental origins. *Monographs of the Society for Research in Child Development, 79*(3), 1–185.

Caspers, K., Yucuis, R., Troutman, B., Arndt, S., & Langbehn, D. (2007). A sibling adoption study of adult attachment: The influence of shared environment on attachment state of mind. *Attachment & Human Development, 9*(4), 375–391.

Cassidy, J., & Marvin, R. (1992). *Attachment organization in three and four year olds: Procedures and coding manual*. Charlottesville: University of Virginia.

Cassidy, J., Woodhouse, S., Sherman, L., Stupica, B., & Lejuez, C. W. (2011). Enhancing infant attachment security: An examination of treatment efficacy and differential susceptibility. *Development and Psychopathology, 23,* 131–148.

Cicchetti, D., Rogosch, F., & Toth, S. (2006). Fostering secure attachment in infants in maltreating families through preventive interventions. *Development and Psychopathology, 18,* 623–649.

Greenberg, M., Speltz, M., DeKlyen, M., & Endriga, M. (1991). Attachment security in preschoolers with and without externalizing behavior problems: A replication. *Development and Psychopathology, 3,* 413–430.

Haltigan, J., Leerkes, E., Supple, A., & Calkins, S. (2014). Infant negative affect and maternal interactive behavior during the still-face procedure: The moderating role of adult attachment states of mind. *Attachment & Human Development, 16*(2), 149–173.

Hoffman, K., Marvin, R., Cooper, G., & Powell, B. (2006). Changing toddlers' and preschoolers' attachment classifications: The circle of security intervention. *Journal of Consulting and Clinical Psychology, 74,* 1017–1026.

Kochanska, G., & Kim, S. (2013). Early attachment organization with both parents and future behavior problems: From infancy to middle childhood. *Child Development, 84*(1), 283–296.

Korfmacher, J., Adam, E., Ogawa, J., & Egeland, B. (1997). Adult attachment: Implications for the therapeutic process in a home visitation intervention *Applied Developmental Science, 1*(1), 43–52.

Levy, K., Meehan, K., Kelly, K., Reynoso, J., Weber, M., Clarkin, J., & Kernberg, O. (2006). Change in attachment patterns and reflective function in a randomized control trial of transference-focused psychotherapy for borderline personality disorder. *Journal of Consulting and Clinical Psychology, 74*(6), 1027–1040.

Main, M., & Goldwyn, R. (1998). *Adult attachment scoring and classification system*. Berkeley: University of California at Berkeley.

Moss, E., Cyr, C., & Dubois-Comtois, K. (2004). Attachment at early school age and developmental risk: Examining family contexts and behavior problems of controlling-caregiving, controlling-punitive, and behaviorally disorganized children. *Developmental Psychology, 40*(4), 519–532.

Moss, E., Dubois-Comtois, K., Cyr, C., St-Laurent, D., & Bernier, A. (2011). Efficacy of a home-visiting intervention aimed at improving maternal sensitivity, child attachment, and behavioral outcomes for maltreated children: A randomized control trial. *Development and Psychopathology, 23,* 195–210.

Routh, C., Hill, J., Steele, H., Elliott, C., & Dewey, M. (1995). Maternal attachment status, psychosocial stressors and problem behaviour: Follow-up after parent training courses for conduct disorder. *Journal of Child Psychology and Psychiatry, 36*(7), 1179–1198.

Scher, A., & Mayseless, O. (2000). Mothers of anxious/ambivalent infants: Maternal characteristics and child-care context. *Child Development, 71,* 1629–1639.

Speltz, M., Greenberg, M., & DeKlyen, M. (1990). Attachment in preschoolers with disruptive behavior: A comparison of clinic-referred and nonproblem children. *Development and Psychopathology, 2,* 31–46.

Speltz, M., DeKlyen, M., & Greenberg, M. (1999). Attachment in boys with early onset conduct problems. *Development and Psychopathology, 11,* 269–285.

Talia, A., Daniel, S., Miller-Bottome, M., Brambilla, D., Miccoli, D., Safran, J., & Lingiardi, V. (2014). AAI predicts patients' in-session interpersonal behavior and discourse: A "move to the level of the relation" for attachment-informed psychotherapy research. *Attachment & Human Development, 16*(2), 192–209.

Toth, S., Rogosch, F., Manly, J., & Cicchetti, D. (2006). The efficacy of toddler-parent psychotherapy to reorganize attachment in the young offspring of mothers with major depressive disorder: A randomized preventive trial. *Journal of Consulting and Clinical Psychology, 74,* 1006–1016.

van den Boom, D. (1994). The influence of temperament and mothering on attachment and exploration: An experimental manipulation of sensitive responsiveness among lower-class mothers with irritable infants. *Child Development, 65,* 1457–1477.

van Ijzendoorn, M., Schuengel, C., & Bakermans-Kranenberg, M. (1999). Disorganized attachment in early childhood: Meta-analysis of precursors, concomitants, and sequelae. *Development and Psychopathology, 11,* 225–249.

Beth Troutman PhD is a Clinical Professor in Psychiatry at the University of Iowa Carver College of Medicine. Her teaching, research, and clinical work has focused on improving parent-child interactions for more than 30 years. She has had a foot in more than one theoretical camp since graduate school, conducting research on parenting self-efficacy, temperament, and attachment theory and disseminating Parent-Child Interaction Therapy (PCIT), a behavioral model for improving parenting.

Chapter 7
What Does Not Kill Me Makes Me Stronger

What does not kill me makes me stronger. (Nietzsche 1888)

Three-year-old Rennie[1] *is referred for treatment as a condition of his continued enrolment in his preschool. The director of the preschool reports Rennie often fails to comply with his teacher's directions and several parents have complained about Rennie bullying or hitting other children. Rennie's parents, Lena and Graham, agree to the preschool director's referral for services in order to avoid Rennie having an expulsion on his record. At the initial evaluation, Lena and Graham list several factors that may contribute to Rennie's difficulty in preschool: (1) his preschool teacher is relatively inexperienced and does not have good control of the classroom, (2) Rennie is ahead of his peers academically and may be bored, (3) Attention Deficit Hyperactivity Disorder (ADHD) runs in their family as both Lena and Graham have a brother with ADHD.*

At the initial evaluation, Lena and Graham indicate Rennie does not exhibit behavior problems at home. On the rare occasion when he misbehaves, his parents discipline him using time-outs in his room. Graham describes his childhood as typical and normal. Lena describes her parents as very loving, stating her childhood was "like a Norman Rockwell painting". Given this description, the therapist is surprised when, later in the intake, Lena describes an incident where she was afraid to tell her mother about getting hurt falling out of a tree for fear of being punished. Lena follows this story with a description of a recent visit from her mother. During this visit, Lena's mother criticized her and Graham's parenting of Rennie, noting her other grandchildren were much better behaved as their parents were "willing to spank". Lena is quick to add she has always respected her mother's honesty and high expectations as it taught her to "stand on her own two feet".

Upon entering the room with his mother at the pre-treatment assessment, Rennie explores the toys in the room and settles down to play with some brightly colored blocks. Lena begins quizzing him about the colors of the blocks which he accu-

[1] This is a fictional account illustrating avoidant dyads and parents with dismissing states of mind.

B. Troutman, *Integrating Behaviorism and Attachment Theory in Parent Coaching*,
SpringerBriefs in Psychology, DOI 10.1007/978-3-319-15239-4_7

Table 7.1 Description of avoidant attachment in infant-parent dyads. (Source: Ainsworth et al. 1978)

Avoidant (A)	Spends majority of time in exploratory behavior but quality of exploration and play is relatively poor. The baby is not distressed during separation when the stranger is present. Ignores parent's return, often by feigning interest in toys. Avoids proximity to mother during reunion
A1	Conspicuous avoidance of parent during reunion. If picked up by parent, tends to look away and not mold to parent
A2	The baby displays some greeting on parent's return but it is mingled with avoidance

rately identifies. When Lena announces that she is leaving after the signal from the therapist, he accepts this without comment. During Lena's absence, he continues building with the blocks. He appears somewhat more relaxed than he did when his mother was in the room and the therapist has the impression he enjoys being able to focus on building without having to name block colors. When Lena reenters, Rennie fails to acknowledge his mother. The therapist might have been convinced Rennie failed to notice his mother's return but she noted an increased flurry of activity around tower-building when his mother walked in the room.

At the pre-treatment DPICS assessment, Rennie incorporates a set of zoo animals in his play by making a zoo for them out of the blocks. Lena begins quizzing Rennie about the names of the animals in the zoo set. When the zoo tower he is building falls down, he becomes frustrated and angry. Lena tells him to rebuild it and suggests strategies to make the base more stable. When told to pick up the toys, he becomes angry, saying he didn't have enough time to play because she messed up his tower.

One aspect of this hypothetical vignette consistent with avoidant attachment and dismissing state of mind is a focus on exploration and achievement. Another feature consistent with this pattern of attachment is the difficulty sharing distress or vulnerability with others. In observed interactions between Rennie and his parents, this presents as Rennie turning away his parents or engaging in impersonal conversation with them when they return following a brief separation. In Lena, this presents as describing her childhood as very loving yet describing interactions with her own mother that appear at variance with this description. Lena's tendency to follow up her discussion of a potentially distressing interaction with her mother by a statement that puts a positive spin on the interaction and emphasizes how it made her stronger is also characteristic of dismissing attachment.

Characteristics of avoidant attachment and dismissing state of mind are described in Tables 7.1 and 7.2. Up to 15 % of infants and pre-schoolers in community samples exhibit an avoidant child-parent attachment (Kochanska and Kim 2013; Moss et al. 2004; van Ijzendoorn et al. 1999). A similar rate of avoidant attachment is seen in preschool-aged children referred for disruptive behavior (Greenberg et al. 1991; Speltz et al. 1995; Speltz et al. 1990).

Table 7.2 Description of avoidant attachment in preschooler-parent dyads. (Source: Cassidy and Marvin 1992)

Avoidant (A)	Child is focused on exploration. Interactions do not seem warm or special
Avoidant ignoring (A1)	During reunion, child ignores parent
Avoidant neutral (A2)	During reunion, child may interact with parent but interactions do not appear relaxed or comfortable

Table 7.3 Rates of avoidant attachment in intervention studies

Population	Model	Rate of avoidant attachment	Reference
Infants in maltreating families (United States) N=137	Child-Parent Psychotherarpy (CPP)	Pre CPP: 6%	Cicchetti et al.2006
		Post CPP: 7%	
	Nurse-Family Partnership (NFP)	Pre NFP: 12%	
		Post NFP: 0	
	Community Standard Care (CS)	Pre CS: 4%	
		Post CS: 18%	
Toddlers of mothers with Postpartum Major Depressive Disorder (United States) N=130	Child-Parent Psychotherapy (CPP)	Pre CPP: 36%	Toth et al. 2006
		Post CPP: 17%	
	Control (Con)	Pre Con: 28%	
		Post Con: 35%	
At-risk Head Start and Early Head Start group (N=65) (United States)	Circle of Security (COS)	Pre COS: 17%	Hoffman et al. 2006
		Post COS: 11%	
First born, irritable infants in economically stressed households (United States) N=220	Circle of Security—Home Visiting-4 Intervention	COS-HV4: 11%	Cassidy et al. 2011
	(COS-HV4)	Con: 17%	
	Control (Con)		

Parenting Behavior Associated with Avoidant Attachment

The parenting behavior associated with avoidant attachment is lack of sensitive responsiveness to infant distress (Ainsworth et al. 1978; van den Boom 1988, 1989, 1994). As seen in Tables 7.3 and 7.4, a parent coaching intervention that improves maternal sensitive responsiveness to infant distress and positive attachment signals in a sample of Dutch, irritable infants is clearly effective in reducing rates of avoidant attachment (van den Boom 1994) while interventions targeting sensitive responsiveness in maltreatment populations do not appear to significantly reduce avoidant attachment in these populations. Given the significant stressors in these populations, it may be difficult for these dyads to overcome a tendency to turn away when they feel vulnerable or distressed once this pattern has been established. Circle of Security protocols which educate parents about secure attachment and

Table 7.4 Rates of avoidant attachment in parent coaching interventions

Population	Model	Rate of avoidant attachment	Reference
First born, irritable, low SES infants (Netherlands) $N=100$ @ 12 mos.; 82 @ 18 mos.	Skills-Based Intervention (SBI) Control (Con)	SBI @ 12 mos.: 24% SBI @ 18 mos.: 19% Con @ 12 mos.: 52% Con @ 18 mos.: 51%	van den Boom 1994
Maltreated infants and preschoolers (French Canadian) ($N=67$)	Relationship Intervention Program (RIP) Community Services (CS)	Pre RIP: 14% Post RIP: 14% Pre CS: 12% Post CS: 6%	Moss et al. 2011

Table 7.5 Characteristics of dismissing state of mind. (Sources: Main and Goldwyn 1998; Steele and Steele 2008)

Dismissing of attachment (Ds)	Dismisses the importance of early attachment relationships by failing to recognize negative early experiences and/or negative effects of difficult early experiences. Generalized descriptions of relationships with parents (semantic level) are not supported by specific memories, attachment figures are devalued, or adult reports he was not affected by early experiences or negative experiences made him stronger
Dismissing of attachment (Ds1)	Discrepancy between generalized picture of parent as excellent or normal and descriptions of childhood interactions that do not support or actively contradict this picture. Insists they have no memory for childhood and presents this as normal
Devaluing of attachment (Ds2)	Parents or attachment-related experiences are described with contempt
Restricted in feeling (Ds3)	Difficult childhood attachment experiences are mentioned but followed by an upbeat description of parents or the positive impact of difficult experiences. Childhood is described as normal or typical but there are no specific memories consistent with this description
Cut-off from the source of fear of death of the child (Ds4)	Fear of child's death that parent fails to connect to any specific source

prompts them to reflect on barriers to responding to their child's attachment signals, are associated with reduced rates of avoidant attachment

Dismissing State of Mind

Characteristics of dismissing state of mind are summarized in Table 7.5. Approximately one-third of adolescents and adults in community samples have a dismissing state of mind (Bakermans-Kranenburg and van Ijzendoorn 2009; Booth-LaForce and Roisman 2014). A similar rate is found in parents participating in parent management treatment for disruptive disorder (Routh et al. 1995), patients receiving psychotherapy for borderline personality disorder, adults who had been adopted as infants (Caspers et al. 2007), foster mothers (Dozier et al. 2001b), and adoptive fathers (Steele et al. 2008). Populations with lower than typical rates of dismissing state of mind (12 to 16 %) include low income mothers participating in a preventive home visiting intervention (Erickson et al. 1992), adoptive mothers (Steele et al. 2008), and parents of children with autism (Seskin et al. 2010).

Research on Dismissing State of Mind

Mothers with dismissing state of mind tend not to attune to their infant's negative affect (Haft and Slade 1989). In a recent study of pregnant women's physiological response (heart rate, skin conductance, and respiratory sinus arrhythmia) to brief video segments of mother-infant interactions, women with a dismissing state of mind exhibit physiological responses associated with aversive consequences when watching a video of a mother unable to soothe her crying infant (Ablow et al. 2013). Surprisingly, watching a video of a mother and infant playing contentedly evokes a similar physiological response. This study helped me realize that while early interventionists typically consider playing with children a positive experience, for parents with a dismissing state of mind it can be akin to nails on a chalkboard.

During individual therapy sessions, adults with dismissing state of mind are less likely to express distress to their therapist, ask for help, or express gratitude to the therapist (Talia et al. 2014). They are more likely to directly avoid the therapist's questions by responding briefly and then becoming silent, downplay distress by laughing after recounting a distressing experience, or disqualify negative feelings by conveying self-sufficiency (Talia et al. 2014). During interactions with their case managers, adults with dismissing state of mind and a diagnosis of schizophrenia or bipolar disorder, spent more time off task (Dozier et al. 2001a). Interestingly, this was due to the case managers changing the topic more frequently, presumably in response to nonverbal cues indicating the person was uncomfortable. During interactions with their significant others, adults with Dismissing state of mind and a diagnosis of schizophrenia or bipolar disorder used more active distancing strategies when sensitive topics were raised, e.g. sighing and making sarcastic comments. The significant others of individuals with dismissing state of mind reported more sadness following problem-solving interactions with their partner.

Clinical Observations and Recommendations

Countertransference Reactions

In dyads with an avoidant attachment/parents with a dismissing state of mind, parents and children tend to be critical of each other and of the provider, leading the provider to feel he needs to protect himself from challenges and criticisms. Parents who drop out of behavioral parenting interventions criticize their child more often during the pre-treatment behavioral assessment than parents who complete treatment (Fernandez and Eyberg 2009) and parent coaches are more critical and directive of parents who criticize their child more during child-led play sessions (Barnett et al. 2014). These two studies remind me that when faced with a parent who frequently criticizes me and their child, I need to remain aware of how this affects me so I am not pulled into a negative cycle. I focus on identifying the parent's strengths so I can give them genuine praise during coaching sessions. (I sometimes need to seek consultation from another therapist in order to identify these strengths and why this parent gets under my skin). I often use the code the coach form in Chap. 4 to evaluate whether I am giving them enough positive feedback during sessions. With preoccupied parents the criticism of the provider tends to be more nattering and whiny (Yes, but) while with dismissing parents it tends to be more pointed and sarcastic (You may have gone to school for a long time but you don't know what you're talking about.)

When I am able to avoid the countertransference trap of returning criticism and sarcasm with criticism and sarcasm, I find myself doing more self-disclosure related to vulnerable feelings with these families. For example, when they describe objectively difficult situations that were "not a big deal" or "made them stronger", I often find myself describing how I have felt in a similar difficult situation. I find Bollas' (1987) writing about the normotic personality (someone who is "abnormally normal") especially useful in understanding this countertransference reaction. Bollas (1987) describes interviewing an adolescent patient who, despite two recent suicide attempts, behaved as a confident, socially skilled young man who acted as though nothing out of the ordinary had happened in the past month. When attempts to understand the patient's experience were deflected with statements about how things would turn out for the best, Bollas begins to describe his own feelings of uncertainty and doubt as an adolescent.

The lack of warmth and positive interactions in avoidant and dismissing dyads can lead providers to wonder whether the child is "unattached". I find it helpful to remember the detachment response of young children to separations first documented by Robertson. The child the parent spent the most time with prior to the separation was the one they turned away from and did not "remember" when reunited with the parents. Avoidance was not an indication that the child was no longer attached to the parent but rather an indication of how difficult it was for them to trust the person they had most depended on when the relationship had been disrupted. Similarly, in avoidant dyads, the child is protecting himself from feeling too close and vulnerable and maintaining the attachment relationship by not being too needy.

I have the most concerns about using behavioral interventions with dyads with avoidant attachment. Specifically, I'm concerned teaching parents to use ignoring and time-outs for their child's misbehavior will reinforce their tendency to turn away from their child's distress. Ironically, I suspect behavioral interventions are more appealing to parents with a dismissing state of mind as the focus is on learning strategies for managing behavior rather than on feelings or relationships.

When working with individuals with a dismissing state of mind, the key concept to remember is deactivation of attachment. They do not like to ask for help so are typically being coached in interactions with their child due to desperate circumstances where they consider the alternative a worse consequence than seeking help. Parents at the more extreme end of the dismissing continuum often enter treatment with a chip on their shoulder and armed with the latest research findings about the best way to address their child's problems. Providers who are themselves a bit dismissing and prone to a sarcastic viewpoint may find themselves thinking "If you're such an expert, why are you here anyway?" Of course, you have the impression the parent would respond to that question with a list of factors that have nothing to do with their parenting. The truth is parents with a dismissing state of mind often experience a great deal of shame about their child's difficulties. However, the idea of acknowledging this to themselves or someone else is excruciating.

Coaching Child-led Play

Parents in avoidant dyads are more comfortable with their child's exploration needs than they are with their attachment needs. However, they also struggle with supporting their child's exploration. They tend to be focused on teaching their child or competing with their child rather than letting their child explore. Also, they become uncomfortable when their child struggles with a task, becomes frustrated, or asks for help. Helping parents in avoidant dyads use behavioral parenting skills to support their child's exploration is often a good first step towards improving attachment security. I often explain the concept of scaffolding to parents to give them a sense of how important they are to their child's ability to explore and learn. I note that just as a scaffold is needed while a building is being constructed but is later taken down, their ability to support their child's completion of a task by describing and praising his efforts facilitates their child's ability to eventually complete the task on his own. The types of toys I have found are best for teaching parents the power of scaffolding are those involving magnets that hold two pieces together (e.g. I have a toy train where the cars are held together by magnets and a magnetic building toy). When I first teach parents behavioral parenting skills they will be using during child-led play, I will role play struggling with trying to put together two magnet ends that repel each other. Parents will invariably tell me how to do it or take the toy from me to show me how to do it (at which point I have a great deal of countertransference information about the experience of being their child!). I then have them practice describing what I'm doing and praising my efforts to stick with the task until I find the two magnet ends that fit together. When this situation comes up when I am coaching child-led play, parents have had some experience practicing a different response to their child's struggles during exploration. When they experience their child's ability to solve this problem with their support, it is typically a powerful moment for both of them.

By the time children with an avoidant pattern of attachment are referred for behavior problems, there is a well-established pattern of both the parent and child turning away from feelings of vulnerability in order to avoid being hurt. Behavioral interventions that focus on increasing positive interactions can be a first step to addressing this pattern by giving the parent and child an opportunity to practice the vulnerability associated with expressing gratitude. In avoidant attachment, the members of the dyad turn away from each other before they have an opportunity to feel vulnerable in order to avoid being hurt. Thus, one of the issues that comes up in these dyads is the child saying they don't want to play with their parent and the child rejecting or mocking their parent's use of behavioral parenting skills. When coaching parents through these moments, it is important to acknowledge how difficult it is for the parent to keep using the skills when their child is rejecting them and to praise them for the courage to keep trying. Parents in these dyads often have a difficult time completing assignments to do child-led play at home. Once they begin completing child-led play at home, parents will tend to substitute educational activities for play and to withhold child-led play as punishment on days the child has been "bad". It is important for the therapist to be empathic to the parent's struggle while continuing to set the expectation the parent try child-led play at home. When parents are in an entrenched pattern of rejection and insist their child will not play with them at home, I sometimes tell the parent to try what I call "stealth child-led play", i.e. just spending a minute or two praising their child and attending to their child's positive behaviors when their child is relaxed and engaged in another activity (often video games). For avoidant dyads, engaging in child-led play when upset can be a difficult but powerful intervention since it goes against their instincts to spend time together and be vulnerable rather than retreat into safety.

When presenting the first phase of treatment, child-led play, to Lena and Graham[1]*, the therapist anticipated they might view the guidelines as an indictment of their current parenting and react defensively. The therapist began to establish herself as a safe haven for Lena and Gramah by commenting on how difficult it must be for them to feel blamed for the problems he was having at school, especially when they had worked so hard to facilitate his cognitive development and ensure he was ready for school. The therapist emphasized Lena and Graham's commitment to their son and their willingness to do things that were difficult for the sake of their son. Since she anticipated Lena and Graham might have difficulty with child-led play, she normalized this by stating upfront a lot of parents found child-led play somewhat uncomfortable and "touchy-feely". The therapist noted a lot of parents found it especially difficult to do child-led play child when their child was having a bad day. She noted when children were angry it was not unusual for them to reject their parent's attempts to interact positively. Based on the initial evaluation, the therapist knew they were interested in discipline strategies and the idea that building a positive relationship would improve Rennie's behavior was inconsistent with their worldview. She addressed this by noting they would learn more effective discipline in the second phase of the treatment but the first phase needed to be complete first in order to build the foundation for the discipline phase. The therapist appealed to the parent's achievement orientation by noting a lot of parents did not complete* *behavioral treatment due to the difficulty in learning and mastering the skills. However, since she was concerned the parent's emphasis on achievement might get in the way of becoming more playful and less task-oriented during child-led play, during coaching she downplayed the mastery criteria and focused on helping them see how much Rennie enjoyed spending time with them. She emphasized the importance of doing child-led play every day, describing it as a way to "hit the reset button" when he was having a bad day by finding ways to be positive with him.*

When coaching the first few sessions of child-led play, the therapist's goal was to make positive, responsive comments 90 to 95 % of the time. Her corrective comments targeted the parenting behaviors most likely to interfere with the child enjoying child-led play (criticism and commands) and focused on giving the parents alternatives to criticizing and commanding (e.g. describing their own play or describing Rennie's play). She normalized the parents' struggles, noting she knew it seemed weird to describe your child's play and most parents struggled with learning this new way of interacting with their child.

Coaching Parent-led Play

When coaching parent-led play with avoidant dyads, one of the goals is helping parents remain empathic while setting limits. While parents with a dismissing state of mind often have difficulty following directions themselves, they are often angry or frustrated about their child's difficulty following directions. It is important the provider be "in charge" during initial parent-led play sessions to ensure the session does not become too punitive and to give the parent the experience of a calm, warm authority figure.

Conclusions

Engaging parents in avoidant dyads and parents with dismissing state of mind in parent coaching can be challenging. Child-led play is especially important for these dyads but the idea of improving relationships through play or sharing tender feelings is foreign to individuals in these dyads. The provider's ability to be genuinely positive, genuine, and human with the parent will allow the parent to begin examining their perspective of interactions.

References

Ablow, J., Marks, A., Feldman, S., & Huffman, L. (2013). Associations between first-time expectant women's representations of attachment and their physiological reactivity to infant cry. *Child Development, 84*(4), 1373–1391.

Ainsworth, M., Blehar, M., Waters, E., & Wall, S. (1978). *Patterns of attachment: A psychological study of the strange situation*. Hillsdale: Erlbaum.

Bakermans-Kranenburg, M., & van Ijzendoorn, M. (2009). The first 10,000 adult attachment interviews: distributions of adult attachment representations in clinical and non-clinical groups. *Attachment & Human Development, 11*(3), 223–263.

Barnett, M., Niec, L., & Acevedo-Polakovich, I. (2014). Assessing the key to effective coaching in parent-child interaction therapy: The therapist-parent interaction coding system. *Journal of Psychopathology and Behavioral Assessment, 36,* 211–223.

Bollas, C. (1987). *The shadow of the object: Psychoanalysis of the unthought known.* New York: Columbia University Press.

Booth-LaForce, C., & Roisman, G. (2014). The adult attachment interview: Psychometrics, stability and change from infancy, and develpmental origins. *Monographs of the Society for Research in Child Development, 79*(3), 1–185.

Caspers, K., Yucuis, R., Troutman, B., Arndt, S., & Langbehn, D. (2007). A sibling adoption study of adult attachment: The influence of shared environment on attachment state of mind. *Attachment & Human Development, 9*(4), 375–391.

Cassidy, J., & Marvin, R. (1992). *Attachment organization in three and four year olds: Procedures and coding manual.* University of Virginia.

Cassidy, J., Woodhouse, S., Sherman, L., Stupica, B., & Lejuez, C. W. (2011). Enhancing infant attachment security: An examination of treatment efficacy and differential susceptibility. *Development and Psychopathology, 23,* 131–148.

Cicchetti, D., Rogosch, F., & Toth, S. (2006). Fostering secure attachment in infants in maltreating families through preventive interventions. *Development and Psychopathology, 18,* 623–649.

Dozier, M., Lomax, L., Tyrrell, C., & Lee, S. (2001a). The challenge of treatment for clients with dismissing states of mind. *Attachment & Human Development, 3*(1), 62–76.

Dozier, M., Stoval, K. C., Albus, K. E., & Bates, B. (2001b). Attachment for infants in foster care: The role of caregiver state of mind. *Child Development, 72*(5), 1467–1477.

Erickson, M., Korfmacher, J., & Egeland, B. (1992). Attachments past and present: Implications for therapeutic intervention with mother-infant dyads. *Development and Psychopathology, 4,* 495–507.

Fernandez, M., & Eyberg, S. (2009). Predicting treatment and follow-up attrition in parent-child interaction therapy. *Journal of Abnormal Child Psychology, 37,* 431–441.

Greenberg, M., Speltz, M., DeKlyen, M., & Endriga, M. (1991). Attachment security in preschoolers with and without externalizing behavior problems: A replication. *Development and Psychopathology, 3,* 413–430.

Haft, W., & Slade, A. (1989). Affect attunement and maternal attachment: A pilot study. *Infant Mental Health Journal, 10*(3), 157–172.

Hoffman, K., Marvin, R., Cooper, G., & Powell, B. (2006). Changing toddlers' and preschoolers' attachment classifications: The circle of security intervention. *Journal of Consulting and Clinical Psychology, 74,* 1017–1026.

Kochanska, G., & Kim, S. (2013). Early attachment organization with both parents and future behavior problems: From infancy to middle childhood. *Child Development, 84*(1), 283–296.

Main, M., & Goldwyn, R. (1998). *Adult attachment scoring and classification system.* Berkeley: University of California.

Moss, E., Cyr, C., & Dubois-Comtois, K. (2004). Attachment at early school age and developmental risk: Examining family contexts and behavior problems of controlling-caregiving, controlling-punitive, and behaviorally disorganized children. *Developmental Psychology, 40*(4), 519–532.

Moss, E., Dubois-Comtois, K., Cyr, C., St-Laurent, D., & Bernier, A. (2011). Efficacy of a home-visiting intervention aimed at improving maternal sensitivity, child attachment, and behavioral outcomes for maltreated children: A randomized control trial. *Development and Psychopathology, 23,* 195–210.

Nietzsche, F. (1888). *Twilight of the idols or how to philosophize with a hammer* (D. F. Ferrer, Trans.). https://archive.org/details/TwilightOfTheIdolsOrHowToPhilosophizeWithAHammer. Accesed 1 Sept 2014.

Routh, C., Hill, J., Steele, H., Elliott, C., & Dewey, M. (1995). Maternal attachment status, psychosocial stressors and problem behaviour: Follow-up after parent training courses for conduct disorder. *Journal of Child Psychology and Psychiatry, 36*(7), 1179–1198.

Seskin, L., Feliciano, E., Tippy, G., Yedloutschnig, R., Sossin, K., & Yasik, A. (2010). Attachment and autism: Parental attachment representations and relational behaviors in the parent-child dyad. *Journal of Abnormal Child Psychology, 38,* 949–960.

Speltz, M., Greenberg, M., & DeKlyen, M. (1990). Attachment in preschoolers with disruptive behavior: A comparison of clinic-referred and nonproblem children. *Development and Psychopathology, 2,* 31–46.

Speltz, M., DeKlyen, M., Greenberg, M., & Dryden, M. (1995). Clinic referral for oppositional defiant disorder: Relative significance of attachment and behavioral variables. *Journal of Abnormal Child Psychology, 23*(4), 487–507.

Steele, H., & Steele, M. (2008). *Clinical applications of the adult attachment interview*. New York: Guilford.

Steele, M., Hodges, J., Kaniuk, J., Steele, H., Hillman, S., & Asquith, K. (2008). Forecasting outcomes in previously maltreated children: The use of the AAI in a longitudinal adoption study. In H. Steele & M. Steele (Eds.), *Clinical applications of the adult attachment interview*. New York: Guilford.

Talia, A., Daniel, S., Miller-Bottome, M., Brambilla, D., Miccoli, D., Safran, J., & Lingiardi, V. (2014). AAI predicts patients' in-session interpersonal behavior and discourse: A "move to the level of the relation" for attachment-informed *Attachment & Human Development, 16*(2), 192–209.

Toth, S., Rogosch, F., Manly, J., & Cicchetti, D. (2006). The efficacy of toddler-parent psychotherapy to reorganize attachment in the young offspring of mothers with major depressive disorder: A randomized preventive trial. *Journal of Consulting and Clinical Psychology, 74,* 1006–1016.

van den Boom, D. (1988). *Neonatal irritability and the development of attachment: Observation and intervention*. (dissertation), University of Leiden.

van den Boom, D. (1989). Neonatal irritability and the development of attachment. In G. Kohnstamm, J. Bates, & M. Rothbart (Eds.), *Temperament in childhood*. (pp. 299–314). Hoboken: Wiley.

van den Boom, D. (1994). The influence of temperament and mothering on attachment and exploration: An experimental manipulation of sensitive responsiveness among lower-class mothers with irritable infants. *Child Development, 65,* 1457–1477.

van Ijzendoorn, M., Schuengel, C., & Bakermans-Kranenberg, M. (1999). Disorganized attachment in early childhood: Meta-analysis of precursors, concomitants, and sequelae. *Development and Psychopathology, 11,* 225–249.

Beth Troutman PhD is a Clinical Professor in Psychiatry at the University of Iowa Carver College of Medicine. Her teaching, research, and clinical work has focused on improving parent-child interactions for more than 30 years. She has had a foot in more than one theoretical camp since graduate school, conducting research on parenting self-efficacy, temperament, and attachment theory and disseminating Parent-Child Interaction Therapy (PCIT), a behavioral model for improving parenting.

Chapter 8
Like a Refugee

Every heart to love will come but like a refugee
Forget your perfect offering.
There is a crack in everything.
That's how the light gets in.
(Cohen 1992)

ANTHEM
Written by Leonard Cohen

Five-year-old Andy[1] *and his mother, Wendy, are referred by their Department of Human Services (DHS) worker due to concerns about Andy's aggression towards Wendy, his noncompliance at school and home, Wendy's lack of parenting skills, and Wendy's failure to set limits. The DHS worker became involved with Andy's family after the police were called to the home due to a physical altercation between Andy's parents, Wendy and Morris.*

During the intake with Wendy, she requests individual play therapy for Andy to address his anger problems and "keep him from growing up to be just like his father". Wendy reports she currently has a no contact order but Morris will be allowed to have supervised visits with Andy. Wendy indicates she is seeing an individual therapist for depression and posttraumatic stress disorder and states her individual therapist agrees play therapy to address Andy's attachment trauma is the best approach. Later during the intake, Wendy indicates her therapist recommended play therapy for Andy several months ago but she had been too busy to find a therapist and schedule an appointment. At the end of the intake, when the therapist tries to assess Wendy's willingness to participate in parent coaching to improve her relationship with Andy, Wendy states she is interested in being coached in how "not to be pushed around by men". However, she also wants Andy

[1] This is a fictional account illustrating a disorganized dyad and parents with an unresolved state of mind.

B. Troutman, *Integrating Behaviorism and Attachment Theory in Parent Coaching*, SpringerBriefs in Psychology, DOI 10.1007/978-3-319-15239-4_8

to see a play therapist and is not sure she has time to take Andy to both appointments given the demands being placed on her by DHS. She would also like Andy to be evaluated for Attention Deficit Hyperactivity Disorder (ADHD). Wendy reports that Andy has been having difficulty in Kindergarten and his teacher thinks he has ADHD. Wendy agrees to sign releases so the therapist can talk with her individual therapist, DHS worker, and Andy's teacher regarding the various concerns about Andy and the different recommendations regarding the best interventions to address Andy's problems.

During the initial mother-child observation, Andy and his mother enter the room and sit down by a box of foam blocks on the floor. Andy begins building a tower. His mother picks up a block and puts it on his tower. Andy yells "No. It doesn't go there." He takes the block off and throws it. His mother says "You need to play nicely. Stop throwing the blocks." Andy knocks the tower over while looking defiantly at his mother. They continue to argue about the tower and Andy's behavior until the signal comes for Andy's mother to leave the room. When the signal comes for Wendy to leave the room, she tells Andy she needs to leave. Andy whines "Why? I want you to stay and play with me." Wendy says "because she says I have to leave" and eventually gets out of the door. Andy opens the door but when the therapist tells him he needs to stay in the room and his mother will be back soon, he sits down by the blocks. He continues to build but appears listless and unfocused. When Wendy returns to the play room, he commands her to sit down beside him. He continues to be bossy and demanding, occasionally adding a "Do it now bitch" if his mother does not immediately comply with his demands. The therapist feels herself getting increasingly tense as the next separation approaches and moves near the door so she can tell Andy to stay in the room after his mother leaves. After giving the signal for Wendy to leave again, there is another long, drawn out argument between Wendy and Andy about her leaving the room. He does not leave the room this time but sits watching the door until she returns. When she returns, he begins angrily grilling her about where she has been.

Child-led play continues along the same lines with Andy telling Wendy what to do and Wendy yelling at Andy to "Behave", "Act nice", and "Stop yelling at me." The therapist finds herself dreading the next standardized situation—parent-led play. When told to have Andy follow her lead, Wendy defiantly tells Andy "You have to play with what I want to play with now. I'm going to make you play with the doll house." Predictably, Andy refuses. His mother then switches tactics and begins pleading with him to play dolls with her. When asked to pick up the toys, Andy picks up a block and throws it near his mother's head. She then looks towards the one-way mirror and plaintively asks "What am I supposed to do?". The therapist enters the room with a flourish and says "I put too many toys in here today! This is a lot to pick up!" She uses this brief distraction to tell Wendy to not worry about picking up the toys. The therapist focuses her attention on what remains of the tower, exclaiming over how tall it is. The therapist continues to pick up other toys but leaves the tower intact. She tells Andy that she will be sure to have the blocks in the room the next time he and his mom come in to play. The therapist tells Wendy that it was useful to observe Andy and she is hopeful she will be able to help them get along better.

When the therapist sees Andy's muscular and heavily tattooed father, Morris, in the waiting room, she has momentary doubts about her goal to include fathers in treatment whenever possible. Morris seemed to have arrived with a chip on his shoulder, telling the therapist about his plan to have his lawyer sue the city for the "trumped up" charges against him and his plans for getting DHS out of his life before they had even left the waiting room. Once they get back to the therapy room, the therapist thanks Morris for coming in to discuss Andy's treatment. She makes it clear that although Andy was referred by DHS, her understanding is that Morris' involvement in Andy's treatment is voluntary. She tells Morris the goal for today's meeting is to get information about his concerns about Andy and family history that might help her better understand how to help Andy. She tells Morris that at the end of today's session they can discuss whether he wants to be involved in further evaluation and treatment.

Morris seems to relax slightly and talks poignantly about how much he misses his "little guy". The therapist finds herself relaxing and chuckles softly to herself at hearing the young brute who had terrorized his mother and almost destroyed her toys as a little guy. Morris describes his concerns about Andy struggling in school. He said he knows Andy is smart and hopes he will go to college but that he needs to learn to apply himself and get along with the teacher. When asked about family history, Morris describes a litany of losses and placements in foster care due to his parents' substance abuse. He describes being beat with a belt in one of the foster homes. He notes that he deserved it for being a "little shit" to his foster father and that it toughened him up and prepared him for the real world. At the end of the interview, Morris agrees to another appointment where the therapist can observe his interactions with Andy if the therapist "can talk that DHS bitch and his mother" into it.

Due to the no contact order in place between Andy's parents, DHS arranges for a worker to transport Andy to the evaluation with his father. When the therapist enters the waiting room, Andy is already happily telling his father about his day at school. When the therapist enters the waiting room and greets Andy and his father, Andy jumps up and begins tugging on his father's hand saying "She has cool toys!". When they enter the play room, Morris points out the one-way mirror to Andy saying "That's how they watch us." The therapist hands the bug-in-the-ear to Morris and reminds him she will be telling him what to do for each of the different situations. Andy goes over to the parking garage and says "Want to play cars with me?" Morris sits in a chair near the parking ramp and box of cars. He grills Andy about the color and make of each car as Andy races them down the parking ramp. When the signal comes for Morris to leave the room, he says "See you later Bud" and walks out. Andy continues to play with the cars. Wildly racing the cars down the ramp progresses to elaborate car crashes causing the therapist to reflect on Andy's interactions with his mother and wonder about her choice of toys this time. When Morris returns following the 5 min separation, Andy looks at his father with a forced smile and says "Yea!! Daddy's back!" Morris sits down next to Andy by the ramp and cars. Andy abruptly gets up and moves over to the blocks saying "I need to build a garage where the cars can get fixed." Morris tells Andy about his recent car problems while Andy builds with the blocks. Andy continues to build quietly for the next 5 min. When the signal is given for Morris to leave again, he says "Stay here" and walks out the door. Andy continues to build with the blocks during the 5 min separation, making an elaborate and carefully balanced structure. The therapist reflects on her surprise that he was capable of this level of sustained attention given his behavior during the observation with his mother. Andy has his back to the door when his father opens it. Andy startles, turns, and says "Look Daddy! I made you a castle!!" His father sits down next to the castle of blocks and pretends to push it over while tauntingly saying "Would it make you mad if I pushed your castle over?" "That's okay. You can push it over if you want" Andy says. "I'm done playing with blocks." Andy gets up and moves to the toy cash register and begins to scan grocery items, occasionally glancing at his father. When Morris is told to tell Andy to choose any activity he wishes and follow his lead, Morris says "What do you want to play with Bud?" "You want me to knock over your castle and you can build it again?" Andy momentarily looks down and says "I want to play grocery store". "OK" Morris says. "How do you play?" Andy explains the rules of grocery store which involve Morris handing him items to ring up. Five minutes later, the therapist tells Morris to switch to parent-led play. Morris says "I want to play demolition now". He knocks over the blocks, inviting Andy to join in the demolition project. The therapist notices the tenseness in her shoulders and realizes she has been both expecting and dreading Morris knocking over Andy's tower ever since Morris pretended to knock it over earlier. Morris tells Andy to build a new castle. Andy promptly starts a new castle, carefully choosing blocks from the pile. After 5 min of rebuilding, Andy has built another fine structure and the therapist finds herself feeling sad for Andy as she gives Morris the direction to have Andy pick up the toys. Andy complies with his father's commands, scrambling around the room to find blocks that made it to the far corners of the room during the "demolition project".

Disorganized Attachment

The parents' and child's traumatization, the mother's depression, and the child's controlling behavior in the hypothetical family described at the beginning of this chapter is consistent with disorganized/controlling attachment and unresolved state of mind. Dyads with disorganized/controlling attachment have made difficult, painful compromises (largely outside of conscious awareness) to maintain an attachment relationship. When I am consulting on dyads similar to the one described above, therapists will sometimes ask me if the child is "unattached". Nothing could be further from the truth. It is because the child is attached to their primary caregivers, and desperate to maintain those attachments, that they have developed problematic patterns of interactions. They are doing the best they can to maintain relationships with caregivers who do not reliably provide a safe haven or secure base. In dyads with disorganized attachment, it is usually possible to determine a secondary pattern of attachment (i.e. secure (B), avoidant (A), or ambivalent/resistant (C)). Dyads classified as disorganized are considered insecure even if the secondary classification is secure[2]. The most common secondary classification seen in disorganized dyads is ambivalent/resistant (46 %) (van Ijzendoorn et al. 1999).

Parent coaching with disorganized/unresolved dyads is daunting, anxiety-provoking, and often discouraging. It is also some of my most rewarding work. It is a privilege to witness the courage of parents and children developing healthier relationships out of a history of pain and brokenness.

I have come to think of disorganized attachment as a cloudy magnifying glass—it both magnifies and obscures aspects of the secondary pattern. The attachment relationship between Andy and Wendy is disorganized/controlling—punitive with a secondary classification of ambivalent/resistant. The ambivalence and resistance characteristic of ambivalent/resistant attachment is magnified while Andy's anxiety is obscured by his controlling behavior. The attachment relationship between Andy and Morris is disorganized/controlling—caregiving with a secondary classification of avoidant. The tendency of young children to seek their parent's approval is magnified while Andy's tendency to turn away from his father when distressed is obscured by his tendency to entertain and appease his father. Both behaviors are indicative of Andy's desire to maintain his attachment relationship with his father while managing his anxiety about the relationship. Interpretation of Andy's interactions with his father is complicated by the reduction in contact between them following the domestic violence incident Table. 8.1.

Table 8.1 Characteristics of disorganized infant-parent attachment in the strange situation procedure. (Source: Main and Solomon 1990)

Behavior	Example
Sequential display of contradictory behavior patterns	Infant cries for parent during separation but turns and moves away from parent at reunion
Simultaneous display of contradictory behavior patterns	Infant cries while avoiding parent by moving away or hiding behind piece of furniture
Undirected, misdirected, incomplete, and interrupted movements and expressions	Infant begins to approach parent but falls prone in huddled posture
Stereotypies, asymmetrical movements, mistimed movements, and anomalous postures	Infant twists hair in parent's presence and does not seek comfort from parent
Freezing, stilling and slowed movements and expressions	In the midst of crying, infant suddenly stops crying, fails to move for 30 s, and appears dazed
Direct indices of apprehension regarding the parent	When parent enters, child jerks back with fearful expression
Direct indices of disorganization or disorientation	Infant approaches stranger with raised arms when parent enters

[2] Dyads with a disorganized/secure attachment classification are considered insecurely attached, a confusing aspect of attachment nomenclature that has led Lyons-Ruth and Spielman (2004) to refer to this group as disorganized-approach.

Disorganized attachment, assessed at 12 to 18 months of age in the Strange Situation Procedure, is associated with aggressive, oppositional, and disruptive behavior at home and school at 2 to 9 years of age, poorer social and cognitive development at 7 years of age, symptoms of posttraumatic stress disorder at 8 ½ years of age, and symptoms of borderline personality disorder at 28 years of age (Carlson et al. 2009; MacDonald 2008; Madigan et al. 2007; Munson et al. 2001; Smeekens et al. 2007; Stams et al. 2002; van Ijzendoorn et al. 1999). In community samples of infants, the rate of disorganized attachment is around 15 % (van Ijzendoorn et al. 1999). Rates are more than twice as high in mothers with perinatal depression (30–40 %) (Troutman and Momany 2012). Rates are 50–90 % in dyads with a maltreating caregiver or identified as at risk for maltreatment (Bernard et al. 2012; Cicchetti et al. 2006; Moss et al. 2011).

Parenting Behaviors Associated with Disorganized Attachment

Initial research on disorganized attachment focused on "fright without solution", i.e. the irresolvable dilemma caused when the person you rely on for comfort and protection is harmful and frightening (Hesse and Main 2000). Subsequent research has identified a number of other parenting behaviors associated with disorganized attachment, summarized in Table 8.2.

Follow-up studies of dyads with disorganized attachment during infancy find that many of these dyads go on to develop a controlling pattern of attachment (Hesse and Main 2000). The child appears to have resolved the dilemma of "fright without solution" by taking charge of the relationship with the parent in either a punitive or caregiving manner. Characteristics of disorganized and disorganized-controlling attachment in preschool-aged children are shown in Table 8.3.

Table 8.2 Parenting behaviors associated with disorganized attachment. (Sources: Beebe et al. 2010; Hesse and Main 2000; Lyons-Ruth and Spielman 2004; Madigan et al. 2007)

Behavior	Examples
Competing or contradictory caregiving strategies	Gently rubbing crying infant's back while saying "Stop that crying right now!"
Failure to regulate infant's fearful arousal	Dog enters room. Baby begins to cry, turns toward mother, and lifts arms towards mother. Mother says "Don't be such a sissy" and pushes baby away
Affective communication errors	Child begins crying and mother laughs
Interference with infant self-regulation	Infant fusses. Infant begins sucking on hand. Mother pulls baby's hand out of their mouth and says "Don't suck on your hand." Baby's fuss escalates to a cry
Frightening child	Father suddenly swoops in on child while growling. Child swats at father and screams

Table 8.3 Characteristics of disorganized-controlling preschool-aged child-parent attachment in the modified strange situation procedure. (Source: Cassidy and Marvin 1992)

Disorganized (D)	During reunion, child displays disordering of expected sequence of behavior, incomplete or undirected movements, confusion or apprehension, dazed or disoriented expression, or depressed affect
Disorganized-Controlling (D)	During reunion, child takes control of the interaction
Controlling-Caregiving	During reunion, child controls parent by helping or entertaining the parent. Child seems overly excited about parent's return—acts overly cheery or "overbright"
Controlling-Punitive	During reunion, child controls parent through punitive or hostile behaviors. Child may refuse to answer the parent or to play with them

In community samples, around 15% of preschool-aged children exhibit disorganized or disorganized-controlling patterns of attachment with their caregivers (Greenberg et al. 1991; Moss et al. 2004; Speltz et al. 1999; Speltz et al. 1990). Rates are considerably higher (around 40%) in preschoolers with clinically depressed mothers (Toth et al. 2006) and preschoolers referred for disruptive behavior (Greenberg et al. 1991; Speltz et al. 1999; Speltz et al. 1990). About 50% of dyads identified as at risk for maltreatment exhibit a disorganized attachment relationship (Bernard et al. 2012; Moss et al. 2011).

Interventions for Disorganized/Controlling Attachment

As shown in Table 8.4, several different interventions based on attachment theory lead to reduction in disorganized/controlling attachment. These interventions share an emphasis on increasing sensitive responsiveness and reducing disorganized caregiving behaviors. Several of these interventions use video feedback to reinforce sensitive responsiveness and help parents reflect on aspects of their behavior that are disorganizing for their child (see Table 8.5.)

Characteristics of Unresolved/Disorganized (u/d) State of Mind

The Adult Attachment Interview (AAI) state of mind associated with disorganized/controlling attachment is unresolved (disorganized/disoriented) (U/d) (Main and Goldwyn 1998; Steele and Steele 2008). Two types of disorganizing/disorienting experiences are assessed by the AAI; loss of an important relationship through death and abuse by an attachment figure. Bowlby notes the loss of an attachment figure

Table 8.4 Rates of disorganized and disorganized/controlling attachment in intervention studies

Population	Model	Rate of disorganized/controlling attachment	Drop-out rate	Reference
Infants in maltreating families (United States) *N*=137	Child-Parent Psychotherapy (CPP) (in home) Nurse Family Partnership (NFP) Community services (CS)	Pre CPP: 88% Post CPP: 32% Pre NFP: 83% Post NFP: 46% Pre CS: 93% Post CS: 78%	CPP: 12% NFP: 8% CS: 33%	Cicchetti et al. 2006
Toddlers of mothers with Postpartum Major Depressive Disorder (United States) N=130	Child-Parent Psychotherapy (CPP) Control (Con)	Pre CPP: 38% Post CPP: 11% Pre Con: 41% Post Con: 41%	CPP: 30% TAU: 13%	Toth et al. 2006
At-risk Head Start and Early Head Start preschool-aged children (United States) *N*=65	Circle of Security (COS)	Pre COS: 60% Post COS: 25%	0	Hoffman et al. 2006
First born, irritable, economically stressed infants (United States) (N=220)	Circle of Security—Home Visiting-4 Intervention (COS-HV4) Control (Con)	COS-HV4: 14% Con: 18%	COS-HV4: 5% Con: 4%	Cassidy et al. 2011

Table 8.5 Rates of disorganized and disorganized/controlling attachment in parent coaching interventions

Population	Model	Rate of disorganized/controlling attachment	Drop-out rate	Reference
First born, irritable, low socioeconomic status (SES) infants (Netherlands) *N*=100 @ 12 mos.; 82 @ 18 mos	Skills-Based Intervention (SBI) Control (Con)	12 mos. Post SBI: 8% Post Con.: 12% 18 mos. Post SBI: 7% Post Con.: 10%	0%	van den Boom 1994
Adopted infants (Netherlands) *N*=98	Video-feedback Intervention to Promote Positive Parenting (VIPP)	Post VIPP: 6% Post Con: 22%	0%	Juffer et al. 2005
Maltreated infants and preschool-aged children (Canada) *N*=66	Relationship Intervention Program (RIP) Community Services (CS)	Pre RIP: 54% Post RIP: 20% Pre CS: 50% Post CS: 56%	RIP: 7% CS: 15%	Moss et al. 2011
Infants and toddlers at risk for maltreatment (United States) *N*=120	Attachment and Biobehavioral Catch-Up (ABC) Developmental Education for Families (DEF)	Post ABC: 32% Post DEF: 57%	0%	Bernard et al. 2012

Table 8.6 Characteristics of unresolved/disorganized/disoriented (U/d) state of mind in the Adult Attachment Interview (AAI). (Sources: Main and Goldwyn 1998; Steele and Steele 2008)

Description	Example
Lapses in the monitoring of reasoning during discussions of a loss	Speaks about someone who is deceased in the present tense as though they are still alive. Speaks as though they caused the death through thoughts or acts that could not have caused death in reality
Lapses in the monitoring of discourse during discussions of a loss	Eulogistic, rehearsed speech when discussing a loss. Prolonged silences when discussing a loss
Report of extreme behavioral reaction to loss	Describes onset of serious substance abuse problem following loss. Describes suicide attempt or hospitalization for depression following loss
Unsuccessful denial of abuse	Describes clear report of abuse at times and denies abuse at other times
Disoriented speech when discussing abuse	Speech becomes markedly incoherent when discussing abuse
Fears of being "possessed" by abuser	Describes fear that physically abusive father will take over her behavior and cause her to abuse her child

is inherently disorganizing and disorienting as the individual has organized their feelings, thoughts, and actions around a specific, important person (Bowlby 1969, 1980). Bowlby defines healthy mourning as accepting the loss of an attachment figure and reorganizing feelings, thoughts, and actions consistent with this change in the real world (Bowlby 1969, 1980). In the AAI, extreme behavioral reactions to the loss of a loved one and lapses in the monitoring of thoughts or discourse that occur more than a year following the death of a loved one are indicators or unresolved/disorganized/disoriented (U/d) attachment. Examples of indicators of unresolved attachment are provided in Table 8.6. Abuse by an attachment figure is inherently disorganizing and disorienting as the person the child is biologically predisposed to go to for comfort and protection is also the source of pain and anxiety. Continuing pain, regret, and sadness about abuse is not considered disorganized or disoriented. In fact, clinical observations suggest parents who are able to remember the pain and sadness associated with abuse by a parent are less likely to abuse their own children (Fraiberg et al. 1975).

The majority of parents (53 %) in a disorganized dyad have an unresolved/disorganized state of mind (Ud) associated with attachment loss, abuse, or trauma (Van Ijzendoorn 1995). Mothers in disorganized dyads have been described as being in a continuing state of fear (Beebe et al. 2010). In community samples, rates of unresolved/disorganized state of mind range from 6 to 25 % (Bakermans-Kranenburg and van Ijzendoorn 2009). Rates among adults adopted as infants and foster mothers are near the top of this range (Caspers et al. 2007; Dozier et al. 2001). Rates are higher among adults seeking parent management training to address their child's conduct problems or psychotherapy services for themselves. In a study of parents participating in parent management training for a child with disruptive behavior, 43 % exhibit unresolved/disorganized state of mind (Routh et al. 1995). 72 % of patients seeking treatment for Posttraumatic Stress Disorder related to childhood abuse (Stovall-McClough and Cloitre 2003) and 32% of patients receiving treatment for Borderline Personality Disorder (Levy et al. 2006) exhibit unresolved/disorganized state of mind.

Research on Unresolved/disorganized State of Mind

In a study of a parenting intervention based on attachment theory, mothers classified as unresolved/disorganized on the AAI were the least likely to engage in problem-solving around parenting tasks (21%) and the most likely to seek crisis intervention (42%) (Korfmacher et al. 1997). Consistent with a crisis orientation to treatment, they participated in fewer sessions than mothers who were not unresolved. Mothers with unresolved state of mind were rated as having less constructive interactions with other partipants and as having more roadblocks to treatment participation. Providers rated their interactions with mothers with unresolved state of mind as more frustrating and less enjoyable (providers were not informed of mother's AAI classification).

Interventions for Unresolved/disorganized State of Mind

Patients who receive Prolonged Exposure (PE) or Skills Training in Affective and Interpersonal Regulation (STAIR) for child-abuse related Posttraumatic Stress Disorder (PTSD) show a significant decrease in unresolved/disorganized state of mind (Stovall-McClough and Cloitre 2003). Controlled exposure to child distress in women with violence-related PTSD leads to a significant reduction in mothers' negative attributions about their child (Schechter et al. 2006). In this study, a therapist explored 4 brief (30 s) video clips with mothers: a moment of optimal parent-child interaction, a moment of separation from mother, a moment of reunion with mother, and a moment of sub-optimal parent-child interaction. After each video clip, the therapist asked a series of questions designed to help the mother reflect on the interaction (e.g. "Tell me what happened." "What were you feeling then?" "What were you feeling as you were watching this moment with me?") (Schechter et al. 2006). These results lead me to conceptualize my parent coaching with disorganized dyads in terms of (1) learning new patterns of interaction and (2) maintaining these new patterns of interaction through gradual exposure to anxiety/stressful situations that are likely to evoke old patterns of behavior for both the parent and child.

Patients with borderline personality disorder who receive a year of Transference-Focused Psychotherapy (TFP), Dialectical Behavior Therapy (DBT), or Supportive Psychotherapy (SPT) fail to show any change in unresolved/disorganized state of mind (Levy et al. 2006).

Clinical Observations and Recommendations

Countertransference

Countertransference responses to disorganized dyads can be like a fun house mirror. Our emotional and behavioral reactions to these dyads can be distorted and extreme. For example, one therapist may find herself viewing the child through the parents' state of mind to such an extent she begins viewing a 4-year-old child as "victimizing" his parent while another therapist may find herself viewing the parent through the child's state of mind to such an extent she views the parent as "mean", "scary", or "incompetent".

I think of observing disorganizing parenting behavior as seeing something out of the corner of your eye. I think the first few times I saw a parent intentionally frighten a child or laugh at a child's distress it was so surprising and disconcerting, I literally turned away. There are still times when the behavior occurs so quickly and I am so taken off guard, I go back and watch the video of the session to ensure I really observed what I think I did.

Framework for Working with Dyads with Disorganized/controlling Attachment

In dyads with disorganized attachment, both the parent and child have difficulty in managing their distress or reaching out to others for assistance in managing distress. Thus, the most important thing to keep in mind in working with disorganized attachment and unresolved/disorganized state of mind is the role of anxiety. I sometimes tell trainees that anxiety is contagious and these are the families that cause providers the most anxiety and stress. The role of anxiety in disorganized attachment and unresolved state of mind and the improvement in unresolved/disorganized state of mind with exposure leads me to conceptualize working with these dyads in terms of controlled exposure approaches for anxiety. Although it is often hard to remember the role of anxiety when hearing a young child call his mother a fucking bitch or observing a mother purposefully tease and frighten her child, these extreme behaviors are typically indicators of anxiety. My first goal when working with these dyads is to make the therapy room a sanctuary. I think of it as a respite from the war zone that is their lives.

On the Adult Attachment Interview (AAI), unresolved state of mind is often not revealed until the part of the interview where the person discusses attachment-related loss or trauma. Similarly, unresolved state of mind is often not immediately obvious in parent coaching. This state of mind is easiest to miss in parents who present as extremely competent in most areas of functioning. In these parents, it is primarily under stress that you see glimpses of the aspects of unresolved state of mind that influence their perceptions of their child. In parents where the unresolved state of mind is a more pervasive aspect of the parent's functioning, I have the impression they are seeing a completely different child or interaction than I see as their perceptions are so distorted by their state of mind.

In keeping with the goal of making your therapy room a sanctuary for the parent and child, be prepared to interrupt the initial observation if you become concerned the child's behavior or parent's behavior is becoming too aggressive or destructive. Since you haven't begun treatment yet, the only goal is to establish yourself and your therapy room as a safe haven. If you have to enter the room due to aggression or destructive behavior, do what you can to distract the parent and child and help them become more regulated. Strategies I have used include: suggesting the parent take a break—e.g. having them walk down the hall and get a drink of water, picking up the toys, doing child-led play with the child, and turning down the lights in the room. Typically, I keep up a running monologue of what I'm doing. I let the parent know I understand the seriousness of the situation by saying I am so glad they have brought their child in for services as I can certainly see the need for these problems to be addressed. In dyads such as the hypothetical mother-child dyad described at the beginning of this chapter, I want to convey both a message of hope and ability to rescue them from the child's aggression (speaking to their state of mind and caregiving pattern) and acknowledgement of their efficacy and competence (letting them know I will not abandon them when they become competent).

Parents with this state of mind and caregiving pattern tend to unconsciously increase or emphasize affect and problems in order to elicit support from you. I find even initial psychoeducational sessions can be surprisingly emotional and parents may become tearful and angry. It is important to acknowledge their affect, be empathic, but keep focused on the goals for the session. It is easy to be pulled into unproductive discussions of affect with parents with unresolved state of mind, especially if they are also preoccupied. You need to convey the sense that you see their affect, are not overwhelmed by it, and know they are capable of parenting despite their affective dysregulation. I often give labeled praises about their ability to parent, make it to the appointment, etc. despite the "week you've had", "your depression", "what's going on in your life", "what you've been through". With parents with unresolved state of mind, I emphasize that this will be a long, hard road but that I am hopeful we will see improvements. Traumatized parents can often not imagine things being different so will not believe you if you are too positive and optimistic. If the child was aggressive during the initial observation, talk about your experience in working with aggressive children. If the child was relatively well-behaved, the parent will likely view this as part of the child being manipulative. Don't contradict them but let them know it is a good sign that the child is capable of behaving appropriately in some situations and that you don't have to see the child's behavior problems in order to believe it. Emphasize how your therapy room and toys are specifically designed to work with children with severe behavior problems so it is unlikely you will ever see problems as severe as the problems seen at home. I do not typically assign homework until I have had an opportunity to coach parents in disorganized dyads as I am concerned it will go very poorly.

Coaching Child-led Play

I find it is helpful to do a couple of minutes of child-led play with the child prior to beginning parent coaching. I do not present this as "modeling" skills for the parent but as an opportunity for me to get to know the child better and for the parent to be able to relax for a couple of minutes. I find beginning with a brief respite for both the parent and child allows them to start off parent coaching on a better foot. Although I typically observe and code at the beginning of each session, I am prepared to terminate coding early if necessary. With this type of dyad, I have seen the parent and child escalate during the first couple of minutes I am out of the room. I want the parent and child to get used to the structure of activities that occur each session but am not rigid about the amount of time I spend coding.

I watch for indicators of caregiver helplessness/being frightened of the child such as flinching, wincing, sitting outside of the child's reach as well as indicators of caregiver hostility and frightening behavior. In the disorganized dyads I work with, I find there is often a mixture of frightened and frightening behavior. Even the most helpless caregivers display brief moments of hostility or frightening behavior. Examples of frightening behavior you might see during child-led play sessions include: teasing the child by taking away a toy or dangling it just out of their reach, teasing the child by poking them with a toy, "stirring the child up" after they have calmed down by "gently" poking them with a toy or object, growling at the child (either directly or, more frequently, through play). See Table 8.4 for further examples of disorganizing parent behavior. When I see these behaviors, it is an indication the parent is becoming anxious and dysregulated. The first time I see the behavior during a child-led play session, I note it to myself and try to coach the parent in activities that will help them calm such as coloring, putting beads together, or doing sewing cards. If I see a second indicator during the session, I will find an excuse to go into the room, send the parent for a break if necessary, and do child-led play with the child.

Either at that session or a session with just the parent, I will talk with the parent about how they appear to feel "constantly on guard" or "walking on eggshells" with their child. I tell them I understand they feel a need to jump in and manage their child's behavior because they know how bad it can get. I find video feedback sessions especially valuable with disorganized dyads as it allows me to gradually expose the parent to the aspects of their child's behavior that are disorganizing for them.

In terms of positive behavioral parenting skills, I find behavior descriptions are typically a good behavioral skill to do first. Parents in disorganized dyads often find using praise challenging as they tend to defend against a positive view of the child. When I first introduce the use of praise to parents in disorganized dyads, I find it helps if I can pair praise of the parent with praise of the child—e.g. he is sticking with that activity because of your great behavioral descriptions. I find acknowledging when I see their child misbehaving also helps establish a more trusting relationship with parents with an unresolved state of mind. I find parents with an extremely negative view of their child are more likely to accept positive statements about their child when they know I am also willing to acknowledge negative aspects of the child.

I find the idea of child-led play is often frightening to parents in disorganized dyads. Their experience of childhood is feeling at the mercy of the adults in their lives and their expectation of child-led play is they will be at the mercy of their child. Therefore, I typically present this phase of treatment as child-led within certain parameters—i.e. child-led when the child is behaving appropriately. Parents in these dyads often worry child-led play will cause the child to become more bossy and controlling. I acknowledge that this is a perfectly reasonable assumption and describe the fact that children become less controlling when they are involved in child-led play as a paradoxical effect of play therapy that is well-known by play therapists.

I tend to have a lower tolerance for child disruptive behavior or aggression—even play aggression - with this type of dyad than I would with other dyads or if I were doing play therapy with the child as I know how quickly anxiety and disorganization can escalate. If the child engages in aggression during child-led play, I tell the parent to give a warning that if they do it again, play will be over. The parent informs the child I will come in and the parent will wait outside for a few seconds. This keeps the aggression from escalating and gives the parent and child a chance to become calmer and more regulated.

During child-led play, I begin to look for opportunities to shape how the child talks to the parent—having the parent ignore instances where the child is bossy and demanding and praise when the child speaks to them appropriately. Sometimes in these dyads, the habit of talking to the parent in a demanding tone of voice is so ingrained you need to find opportunities outside of the parent-child interaction to praise an appropriate tone of voice—e.g. praising tone of voice when the child is pretending to be a character in play.

I begin to challenge the parent's perception of helplessness by making observations to the parent about instances when the child needs them or wants their approval. E.g. "He is showing you what he made. He really wants your approval." Later on during child-led play, I may begin to gently challenge the parent's state of mind. For example, during a sweet moment when the child has crawled up into his mom's lap or has made something for her "He seems so little right now. It is easy to forget how little he is when he is acting like a tough guy most of the time."

After I have established a good therapeutic alliance with parents in disorganized dyads, I begin addressing the indicators of helpless/hostile caregiving. Initially, I just point them out to make the parent aware of them and aware that I see them. For example, I might say "It looks like it frightened you a little when he crashed those blocks."

Children with a disorganized/controlling attachment style become more controlling when they become more anxious—especially when they become anxious about their parent's availability. Ironically, they often become more controlling when the parent begins doing child-led play or praising them—saying "Stop that." or "Don't do that" in response to the caregiver's efforts. The child has developed a strategy for managing the unpredictability of caregivers. Thus, changes in the interaction, even positive changes, evoke anxiety, their working model of a need to control the interaction, and their behavioral strategy of trying to control the caregiver. This, in turn, triggers the parent's feelings of anxiety and helplessness. The combined anxiety of the parent and child may also trigger the parent coach's feelings of anxiety and helplessness, especially the first time the therapist encounters a child who does not respond to child-led play the way they are "supposed to respond".

One of the things I like about the Helping the Noncompliant Child (McMahon and Forehand 2003) protocol is how transparent it is with children about the skills their parents are being taught to use during child-led play. I find this type of transparency is very useful with children in disorganized dyads. In order to help reduce the anxiety about change, I let the child know about the skills I am teaching their parent to use and what will happen if they are aggressive or destructive during child-led play. I also talk about the focus of each child-led play session in front of the child. For example, if I was going to focus on behavioral descriptions during child-led play I might say something like the following to the parent "Remember that during special play today, I want you to describe what he is doing—that lets him know you are seeing him and that what he does is important to you. It is important that he speak respectfully to you. If he is disrespectful, I want you to turn, pick up a toy, and play by yourself until he is ready to play with you. It is also important that everyone plays safely in my room. If he does anything dangerous or destructive, I will come in and play and you will need to wait outside briefly."

Coaching Parent-led Play

Parent-led play is often especially anxiety-provoking for the child and parent in disorganized dyads. Given this knowledge, I provide additional support for both the child and parent during these sessions. For the child, the support involves additional modeling and practice in the procedures of parent-led play (e.g. modeling and practicing walking to the time-out chair). Sometimes, I also use additional rewards (e.g. stickers or hand stamps) for learning to follow directions and take time-outs. For parents, I discuss emotional regulation strategies they find useful and ask them what it will be helpful for them to hear from me during the parent-led play sessions. For these dyads, the return to child-led play after the child has complied or taken a time-out is especially important as it helps both the parent and child calm down and become more regulated.

Conclusions

Coaching someone to become a better parent is a humbling experience. I feel fortunate to be able to draw on research on attachment theory and behaviorism as well as the clinical wisdom of my mentors and trainees in this important work.

Recognizing how much we still have to learn despite how far the science of parenting has advanced, I end with the words of Mary Ainsworth whose writings have taught me so much about the type of researcher, clinician, and person I would like to be. "Science has been so successful that we have arrogant expectations of it; and yet the practical answers, especially, are slow to come. In matters such as rearing an infant—a matter which is of immediate and urgent concern to his parents—it would indeed be good if all the answers were known. They are not—and therefore parents also, and perhaps especially, must have tolerance of uncertainty and be content to do the best they can with the information they have available to them." (Ainsworth 1967)

References

Ainsworth, M. (1967). *Infancy in Uganda*. Baltimore: Johns Hopkins Press.

Bakermans-Kranenburg, M., & van Ijzendoorn, M. (2009). The first 10,000 adult attachment interviews: Distributions of adult attachment representations in clinical and non-clinical groups. *Attachment & Human Development, 11*(3), 223–263.

Beebe, B., Jaffe, J., Markese, S., Buck, K., Chen, H., Cohen, P., Bahrick, L., Andrews, H., Feldstein, S. (2010). The origins of 12-month attachment: A microanalysis of 4-month mother-infant interaction. *Attachment & Human Development, 12*(1), 3–141.

Bernard, K., Dozier, M., Bick, J., Lewis-Morrarty, E., Lindhiem, O., & Carlson, E. (2012). Enhancing attachment organization among maltreated children: Results of a randomized clinical trial. *Child Development, 83*(2), 623–636.

Bowlby, J. (1969). *Attachment and loss. Vol 1: Attachment*. New York: Basic Books.

Bowlby, J. (1980). *Attachment and loss: Vol. 3. Loss*. New York: Basic Books.

Carlson, E., Egeland, B., & Sroufe, L. A. (2009). A prospective investigation of the development of borderline personality symptoms. *Development and Psychopathology, 21*, 1311–1334.

Caspers, K., Yucuis, R., Troutman, B., Arndt, S., & Langbehn, D. (2007). A sibling adoption study of adult attachment: The influence of shared environment on attachment state of mind. *Attachment & Human Development, 9*(4), 375–391.

Cassidy, J., & Marvin, R. (1992). *Attachment organization in three and four year olds: Procedures and coding manual*. Charlottesville: University of Virginia.

Cassidy, J., Woodhouse, S., Sherman, L., Stupica, B., & Lejuez, C. W. (2011). Enhancing infant attachment security: An examination of treatment efficacy and differential susceptibility. *Development and Psychopathology, 23*, 131–148.

Cicchetti, D., Rogosch, F., & Toth, S. (2006). Fostering secure attachment in infants in maltreating families through preventive interventions. *Development and Psychopathology, 18*, 623–649.

Cohen, L. (1992). Anthem. [Recorded by Leonard Cohen] On The Future [CD]. Nashville: Sony.

Dozier, M., Stoval, K. C., Albus, K. E., & Bates, B. (2001). Attachment for infants in foster care: The role of caregiver state of mind. *Child Development, 72*(5), 1467–1477.

Fraiberg, S., Adelson, E., & Shapiro, V. (1975). Ghosts in the nursery: A psychoanalytic approach to impaired infant-mother relationships. *Journal of the American Academy of Child Psychiatry, 14*, 387–421.

Greenberg, M., Speltz, M., DeKlyen, M., & Endriga, M. (1991). Attachment security in preschoolers with and without externalizing behavior problems: A replication. *Development and Psychopathology, 3*, 413–430.

Hesse, E., & Main, M. (2000). Disorganized infant, child, and adult attachment: Collapse in behavioral and attentional strategies. *Journal of the American Psychoanalytic Association*, *48*(4), 1097–1127.

Hoffman, K., Marvin, R., Cooper, G., & Powell, B. (2006). Changing toddlers' and preschoolers' attachment classifications: The circle of security intervention. *Journal of Consulting and Clinical Psychology, 74*, 1017–1026.

Juffer, F., Bakermans-Kranenburg, M. J., & van Ijzendoorn, M. H. (2005). The importance of parenting in the development of disorganized attachment: Evidence from a preventive intervention study in adoptive families. *Journal of Child Psychology and Psychiatry, 46*(3), 263–274.

Korfmacher, J., Adam, E., Ogawa, J., & Egeland, B. (1997). Adult attachment: Implications for the therapeutic process in a home visitation intervention. *Applied Developmental Science, 1*(1), 43–52.

Levy, K., Meehan, K., Kelly, K., Reynoso, J., Weber, M., Clarkin, J., & Kernberg, O. (2006). Change in attachment patterns and reflective function in a randomized control trial of transference-focused psychotherapy for borderline personality disorder. *Journal of Consulting and Clinical Psychology, 74*(6), 1027–1040.

Lyons-Ruth, K., & Spielman, E. (2004). Disorganized infant attachment strategies and helpless-fearful profiles of parenting: Integrating attachment research with clinical intervention. *Infant Mental Health Journal, 25*(4), 318–335.

MacDonald, H., Beeghly, M., Grant-Knight, W., Augustyn, M., Woods, R., Cabral, H., Rose-Jacobs, R., Saxe, G., & Frank, D. (2008). Longitudinal association between infant disorganized attachment and childhood posttraumatic stress symptoms. *Development and Psychopathology, 20*, 493–508.

Madigan, S., Moran, G., Schuengel, C., Pederson, D., & Otten, R. (2007). Unresolved maternal attachment representations, disrupted maternal behavior and disorganized attachment in infancy: Links to toddler behavior problems. *Journal of Child Psychology and Psychiatry, 48*(10), 1042–1050.

Main, M., & Goldwyn, R. (1998). *Adult attachment scoring and classification systems*. Berkeley: University of California.

Main, M., & Solomon, J. (1990). Procedures for identifying infants as disorganized/disoriented during the Ainsworth strange situation. In M. Greenberg, D. Cicchetti, & E. Cummings (Eds.), *Attachment in the preschool years: Theory, research, and intervention*. Chicago: The University of Chicago Press.

McMahon, R., & Forehand, R. (2003). *Helping the noncompliant child: Family-based treatment for oppositional behavior* (2nd ed.). New York: Guilford.

Moss, E., Cyr, C., & Dubois-Comtois, K. (2004). Attachment at early school age and developmental risk: Examining family contexts and behavior problems of controlling-caregiving, controlling-punitive, and behaviorally disorganized children. *Developmental Psychology, 40*(4), 519–532.

Moss, E., Dubois-Comtois, K., Cyr, C., St-Laurent, D., & Bernier, A. (2011). Efficacy of a home-visiting intervention aimed at improving maternal sensitivity, child attachment, and behavioral outcomes for maltreated children: A randomized control trial. *Development and Psychopathology, 23*, 195–210.

Munson, J., McMahon, R., & Spieker, S. (2001). Structure and variability in the developmental trajectory of children's externalizing problems: Impact of infant attachment, maternal depressive symptomatology, and child sex. *Development and Psychopathology, 13*, 277–296.

Routh, C., Hill, J., Steele, H., Elliott, C., & Dewey, M. (1995). Maternal attachment status, psychosocial stressors and problem behaviour: Follow-up after parent training courses for conduct disorder. *Journal of Child Psychology and Psychiatry, 36*(7), 1179–1198.

Schechter, D., Myers, M., Brunelli, S., Coates, S., Zeanah, C., Davies, M., Grienenberger, J. F., Marshall, R. D., McCaw, J. E., Trabka, K. A., & Liebowitz, M. (2006). Traumatized mothers can change their minds about their toddlers: Understanding how a novel use of videofeedback supports positive change of maternal attributions. *Infant Mental Health Journal, 27*(5), 429–447.

Smeekens, S., Riksen-Walraven, J., & van Bakel, H. (2007). Multiple determinants of externalizing behavior in 5-year-olds: A longitudinal model. *Journal of Abnormal Child Psychology, 35*, 347–361.

Speltz, M., Greenberg, M., & DeKlyen, M. (1990). Attachment in preschoolers with disruptive behavior: A comparison of clinic-referred and nonproblem children. *Development and Psychopathology, 2*, 31–46.
Speltz, M., DeKlyen, M., & Greenberg, M. (1999). Attachment in boys with early onset conduct problems. *Development and Psychopathology, 11*, 269–285.
Stams, G., Juffer, F., & van Ijzendoorn, M. (2002). Maternal sensitivity, infant attachment, and temperament in early childhood predict adjustment in middle childhood: The case of adopted children and their biologically unrelated parents. *Developmental Psychology, 38*(5), 806–821.
Steele, H., & Steele, M. (2008). *Clinical applications of the adult attachment interview*. New York: Guilford.
Stovall-McClough, K., & Cloitre, M. (2003). Reorganization of unresolved childhood traumatic memories following exposure therapy. *Annals of the New York Academy of Sciences, 2008*, 297–299.
Toth, S., Rogosch, F., Manly, J., & Cicchetti, D. (2006). The efficacy of toddler-parent psychotherapy to reorganize attachment in the young offspring of mothers with major depressive disorder: A randomized preventive trial. *Journal of Consulting and Clinical Psychology, 74*, 1006–1016.
Troutman, B., & Momany, A. (2012). Use of selective serotonin reuptake inhibitors during pregnancy and disorganised infant-mother attachment. *Journal of Reproductive and Infant Psychology, 30*(3), 261–277.
van den Boom, D. (1994). The influence of temperament and mothering on attachment and exploration: An experimental manipulation of sensitive responsiveness among lower-class mothers with irritable infants. *Child Development, 65*, 1457–1477.
Van Ijzendoorn, M. (1995). Adult attachment representations, parental responsiveness, and infant attachment: A meta-analysis on the predictive validity of the adult attachment interview. *Psychological Bulletin, 117*(3), 387–403.
van Ijzendoorn, M., Schuengel, C., & Bakermans-Kranenberg, M. (1999). Disorganized attachment in early childhood: Meta-analysis of precursors, concomitants, and sequelae. *Development and Psychopathology, 11*, 225–249.

Beth Troutman PhD is a Clinical Professor in Psychiatry at the University of Iowa Carver College of Medicine. Her teaching, research, and clinical work has focused on improving parent-child interactions for more than 30 years. She has had a foot in more than one theoretical camp since graduate school, conducting research on parenting self-efficacy, temperament, and attachment theory and disseminating Parent-Child Interaction Therapy (PCIT), a behavioral model for improving parenting.

Index

B. Troutman, *Integrating Behaviorism and Attachment Theory in Parent Coaching*, SpringerBriefs in Psychology, DOI 10.1007/978-3-319-15239-4

45179164R00081

Made in the USA
Lexington, KY
19 September 2015